Live Longer And Healthier

Ways to Live a Good Life

HANNA AUSTIN

© Copyright 2019 by Hanna Austin

All rights reserved.

This eBook is provided with the sole purpose of providing relevant information on a specific topic for which every reasonable effort has been made to ensure that it is both accurate and reasonable. Nevertheless, by purchasing this eBook you consent to the fact that the author, as well as the publisher, are in no way experts on the topics contained herein, regardless of any claims as such that may be made within. As such, any suggestions or recommendations that are made within are done so purely for entertainment value. It is recommended that you always consult a professional prior to undertaking any of the advice or techniques discussed within.

This is a legally binding declaration that is considered both valid and fair by both the Committee of Publishers Association and the American Bar Association and should be considered as legally binding within the United States.

The reproduction, transmission, and duplication of any of the content found herein, including any specific or extended information will be done as an illegal act regardless of the end form the information ultimately takes. This includes copied versions of the work both physical, digital and audio unless express consent of the Publisher is provided beforehand. Any additional rights reserved.

Furthermore, the information that can be found within the pages described forthwith shall be considered both accurate and truthful when it comes to the recounting of facts. As such, any use, correct or incorrect, of the provided information will render the Publisher free of responsibility as to the actions taken outside of their direct purview. Regardless, there are zero scenarios where the original author or the Publisher can be deemed liable in any fashion for any damages or hardships that may result from any of the information discussed herein.

Additionally, the information in the following pages is intended only for informational purposes and should thus be thought of as universal. As befitting its nature, it is presented without assurance regarding its prolonged validity or interim quality. Trademarks that are mentioned are done without written consent and can in no way be considered an endorsement from the trademark holder.

Table of Contents

INTRODUCTION

You chose this book because you want to change the direction of your life. Though there are many books on this topic, <u>Live Longer and Healthier</u> spoke to. And I am glad it did.

I wrote this book because I wanted to help people. We all have finite lives, but that is no reason to do all we can to live the longest, fullest lives possible. But this is hard to do when you're not raised with the *how* of living such a life. Many of us are raised with one eye on the daily grind and the other on old habits. And, many times, these old habits don't really serve the purpose they once did. Or, worse yet, they became habits based on bad information and have never been much of a service at all.

<u>Live Longer and Healthier</u> takes this into account. It is broken down into six chapters, each covering one common area of life that people want to change. Within each chapter are several smaller sections that break down the why and how of changing each particular part of your life.

You might see a chapter title or the title of a subsection and think it's silly or that it won't apply to you. In order to get the full benefit of

Live Longer and Healthier, I ask that you read each section. I also ask that you give each suggestion a try, even if it seems ridiculous at the time. The tips in this book are based on the changes and choices that helped me and many were and formulated based on the psychology and science behind how we form habits, make changes, and the things that improve our lives.

The book begins with *Reflection and Meditation*. This chapter will help you determine where you're starting from and the changes you want to make. Then, through an easy writing exercise, you will develop a general plan to help achieve your goals. The chapter also contains a few guided meditations and thought exercises to help silence the critic in the back of your head. Used together, these tactics will help support you in making the changes you want to see in your life.

Chapter two covers learning and education. In this book, the terms are used to mean two different concepts, one being the idea of seeking knowledge for its own sake and the other being a formal approach to learning. One key to a happy life is a stimulated mind. And chapter two will help you find your ideal method to keep your mind active.

Once your mind is active, chapter three will help you get your body in gear. It doesn't matter if you've never been an active person or if you already run marathons. There is something here for nearly everyone. It is important to note that chapter two is not a chapter on weight loss or body image. Rather, it is on the positive impacts that physical activity has on our body and different ways you can incorporate more activity into your day. Similarly, chapter four is on the importance of nutrition for the sake of health, rather than weight loss.

Chapters five and six round out the book with a focus on caring for others and for yourself. Humans are social creatures, meaning we seek connection with other people. And, once we leave school, this becomes harder to manage. Chapter five will help you pinpoint ways you might find new friends. Chapter six, on the other hand, will help you learn to befriend yourself.

You only have one mind and one body, after all. Taking care of yourself is the only way to live longer and live healthier.

CHAPTER 1
REFLECTION AND MEDITATION

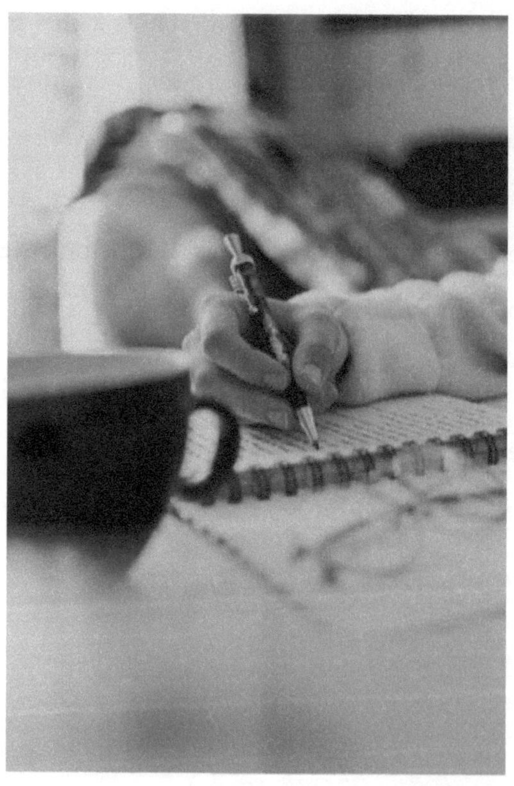

You want to change the way your life is going. If you didn't, you wouldn't be reading this book. But change is often easier to think about than bring about. You've probably experienced this yourself, with failed New Years' resolutions if nothing else. These changes usually fail because there is no framework in place to support. So, before you dive into the external changes this book suggests, you need to make some internal changes.

Acknowledging Your Starting Point

Everything – and everyone – has a beginning. The changes you have in mind are no different. In order to make those changes a reality, you need to acknowledge your starting point. Not an idealized point in the future, either. No, you need to identify the actual place you're starting from.

Your starting point will not look like anyone else's. And that's a good thing. It means that nobody else can make your changes as well as you can. And it means that you can learn and grow at your own pace without comparing yourself to someone else.

Many people struggle to identify their personal starting point. And this can be for a number of reasons. They might not know the general direction they want to go. Or they might have had many false starts in the past and judge themselves on where they think they should be "by now". Most often, however, people struggle to really look at themselves.

Self-reflection can be very difficult, especially when we're reflecting on things we want to change. Looking at where we are now reminded us of how far we have to go. And, for some, it is a reminder that they waited as long as they did to start. But there is no need for this negative self-talk. There is no shame in waiting to make a change or in trying several times to make a change.

So, look at where you're starting. But don't do it with the intent to judge yourself. Instead, look at your starting point as a place of potential. From this moment, you can choose to take yourself in any number of directions. Remind yourself that you cannot change the past. But you can change the rhythm of your life to affect the future.

Choosing a Direction

There are many ways you can choose to change your life, many of which are covered in the following chapters. All of these changes have the potential to help you live longer and to enjoy those additional years as much as possible.

But making a lot of changes all at once will lead to burn out. This is why you should choose one change to make and create a plan. Once those changes are second nature, you can move on to the next change, confident that all of your changes are firmly rooted.

Picking one direction can be overwhelming in and of itself, however. This is why this section contains a writing exercise that should help you prioritize the type of changes you most want to make. The exercise breaks down into two parts, the first of which will help you determine the general category of change you want to see. Once you know the category, part two will help you choose two or three specific changes to make. So, grab a pen, some paper, and a quiet spot so you can get started

First, I want you to imagine your ideal self. You can make this mental image as fanciful as you like. Reject any sense of embarrassment or self-judgment you might feel. This mental image is for you and you alone, so there is no right or wrong answer.

When the image is clear in your mind, write down the first ten things you notice about your ideal self. Are you in a band? Is your hair a wild color? Do you have more confidence in the kitchen? Have you taken up some sport or hobby you've always been too nervous to try? Whatever those first ten details are, write them out.

Now, using those ten details, break them down int0 categories that correspond to the chapters of this book: learning, physical fitness, nutrition, social connections, and self-care. Hobbies and the like would fall under the category of "learning", even if thc hobby involves something in the other four categories.

One of those categories is going to have more in it than the others. This category is the one you're going to focus on first. Before you jump to that chapter, however, you need to set a few specific goals and get a handle on compassionate thinking that will support you as you make strides towards those goals.

To set the specific goals, look at the details you wrote for your category. If, for example, you want to learn a hobby, there are a few steps you'll have to take before you jump right in. You might need to buy supplies, find a class, or clear some time in your schedule. These smaller steps will form the basis for your action plan.

Once you have those steps – now your goals – written down, find a safe place to keep them. You'll want to refer back to them now and then to keep yourself on-track. They will help guide you by reminding you of your ideal self and the steps you're taking to make your ideal your reality.

With your action plan in hand, you might be tempted to jump right into your changes. But if you're still thinking the way you did when you made your last attempts at change, you will run into the same pitfalls. So, before you flip to the chapter that matches your goals, read through the rest of this chapter. It will help you learn compassionate thinking, both for yourself and others, that will make your path a little easier. You will also learn a few guided meditation exercises that you can return to when you need to focus your thoughts and remind yourself why you're on the path you're on.

Creating Compassionate Thinking

You have a critic living in your head. Everyone does. Sometimes that critic can be very helpful. But, most of the time, it is just that: a critic. It tells us what we're doing wrong without offering any insight on how to help. It does not analyze. It does not inform. It just breaks you down.

That voice is not going to get you very far when you're trying to change yourself. Change is messy and it is hard. You're going to fall down and fail. When that happens, you need a cheerleader in your head. Or, at the very least, someone who can see where you went wrong and offer gentle corrections so you can try again. The last thing you need is to tear yourself down with your own thoughts. And that is where compassionate thinking comes in.

Compassionate thinking might sound odd to you. You've heard of compassion, of course. And you know why you need to have compassion for other people. But not many people talk about the need to have compassion for ourselves. Without it, our thoughts just tear us down. And that's not good for our mental health or our chances of success, no matter what we're doing.

Negative self-talk also increases our stress levels, which in turn increase our cortisol levels. And high cortisol levels have been linked to all sorts of nasty things from depression to excess belly fat to heart disease. Changing your inner monologue is a good first step to keeping your cortisol at a more manageable level.

If you're like I was before I learned to think of myself with compassion, your inner critic is screaming right now. It is telling you all sorts of things about how you can't change the voice in your head or that you need someone to "keep you in check" or give you "a dose of reality". To your critic I say – as I had to say to my own – I can do all of that with compassion.

Thinking of yourself with compassion is not code for "never checking your negative behaviors". It is not a full pass to do or think whatever you want, or to ignore reality in favor of a fiction that suits your desires. Instead, it is a push to check in with yourself and to acknowledge reality – good and bad – without berating yourself in the process.

When you apply compassionate thinking to your attempts at change, you put your attempts in a new light. A good example is looking ahead to a time when you will lapse back into old habits. And, until your new behaviors are set as habits, this will certainly happen. When it does, your inner critic will have something nasty to say. "Why even bother, you failed!" is a common thought from an inner critic. Another is "You might as well give up; you obviously can't do it". Even if your inner critic isn't encouraging you to give up, it may be calling you nasty names or belittling you for "failing".

All of these thoughts are wrong. But it can be very hard to acknowledge this when that kind of pressure is coming from inside your own mind. Compassionate thinking, however, frames your relapse in a very different light. Rather than saying "you failed", compassionate thinking says "You made a mistake, but you can get back on track. This behavior won't help you reach your goal, so we'll try to do better next time."

You might already have some fairly compassionate self-talk. Instead of berating yourself for failure, you might good-naturedly call yourself a butterfingers or a nerd. As long as it's thought with a fairly positive tone, these thoughts still count as positive self-talk.

If you're working with more aggressively negative self-talk, however, there are steps you can take to change your inner monologue. The first step is to recognize that it is not acceptable to talk to yourself like that. Not because I said it's not. But because nobody – not even you – should get to talk to you like that. If you would not accept that tone from a friend, a coworker, or a stranger on the sidewalk, you should not accept it from yourself.

You might have to repeat that fact to yourself a few times. That you are worth respect, even – if not more so – from yourself. But the more you repeat it, the more it will set in as a fact. And when it does, you'll find your inner monologue takes on a much more realistic and compassionate tone.

The Styles and Benefits of Meditation

When I say meditation, a whole scene probably popped into your head. Someone is murmuring a soft chant while either gentle music or a sparse yet rhythmic gong sounds in the distance. You probably imagine yourself sitting still on the floor, your thoughts at perfect peace.

This is certainly one version of meditation. But if that doesn't appeal to you – or if you're not sure you can "empty your thoughts" as some meditation practices suggest – there are plenty of different meditation options. The benefits for each vary, but there are a few that span every type of meditation. And all of the benefits, widespread or style-specific, can help you lead a longer, happier life.

The most common meditation benefit is a deeper sense of calm. You've probably heard that you must "clear your mind" when you meditate, but that's not entirely true. Meditation is more about letting your thoughts come and go without getting too hung up in them. Developing this skill allows you to find moments of calm in an otherwise stressful day. And, when you can do this with practiced ease, it leaves you with an outlook that is, overall, much more peaceful.

Meditation also lets you get a better sense of yourself. We all have a thousand thoughts a second. And some of us feel like we have even more. This can be a blessing, allowing us to make connections and fuel creativity at awe-inspiring rates. But it can also leave us drained or unsure of which direction our thoughts were going and why they were going there.

When we meditate, we don't have to follow the tracks our thoughts are on. We can let them come and go, which allows us more of a "bird's eye view" of the way our mind works and what sort of thoughts it seems more preoccupied with. So, when you're plugging away at something for work, you won't be so surprised when a sudden thought about an upcoming event or you're your favorite book or a random song lyric interrupts your workflow. You'll already know your mind is hooked on that subject.

Meditation also gives you the ability to actively let thoughts go. When you're working and that errant thought bursts in, meditation gives you the tools to send it on its way. And, instead of getting frustrated with yourself for losing focus, your compassionate self-talk will kick in to get you back on track and assure you that the thought can be brought back later. Instead of feeling outside of your own mind's inner workings, you'll feel more in control of them.

When you feel more in control of your thoughts and more at peace with the way your thoughts move, you'll find yourself feeling less stressed. Even people with anxiety report reduced symptoms thanks to meditation. They find that their meditation practice gives them the tools to sit down and analyze their thoughts, then let them go to find peace between thoughts. When they do this, the physical symptoms of their anxiety decrease. They might still have anxious thoughts and some physical symptoms. But, overall, they feel less afraid and more prepared to handle their thoughts.

Most meditation is done while sitting still. You either lie on your back or sit in a comfortable position. But those are not your only options. Once you know *how* to meditate, you'll find you can do it anywhere. You could even meditate while floating in a pool if you do it safely.

Those experienced in meditation may even find moving meditation beneficial. This variety of meditation allows you to get up and move, either to music or simply following the whim of your body. It is an excellent option for people who feel restless or hyperactive. It allows them all the benefits of sitting meditation while also allowing their bodies to move as they need to. This approach of two-fold compassion not only puts them more in touch with the way their mind works but also the way their bodies need to move and feel stimulated.

Just as there is a meditation form for people who struggle to sit still, there are also meditation forms for people who need either visual or auditory stimulation. If you are someone who cannot concentrate – while awake – without something to distract your eye, you might find incense or candle flames helpful.

You've probably seen a movie or two where someone stares into the fire or a candle flame as they recount a memory or collect their thoughts. This is a form of meditation and it may work for you too. Incense allows your eyes to track the smoke and notice the way the ember at the tip of the stick smolders and flares. Candles, on the other hand, allow you to watch the dancing of the flame, the melting of the wax, and the way the air moves just below the bell of the flame where it burns so hot, we cannot even see the fire.

If you prefer auditory stimulation, try finding a website that lets you create your own ambient mix. Popular ones include rainstorms, train rides on rainy days, or nights in a country cabin. Many sites with this feature have a wide range of sounds to choose from, up to and including instrumental music. You can create a mix that offers the stimulation you need without distracting you from your meditation.

Meditating with your eyes open or with music playing might seem to undermine the idea of sitting alone with your thoughts. But these options trace back to the idea of having more compassion for yourself. By acknowledging your needs and where you are increasing your odds of success. And, as with compassionate self-talk, giving yourself room to grow from your actual starting point – rather than some fictional point where you think you "should be" to start meditating – reduces your overall stress levels.

There is always some way to meditate and still meet your particular needs. You might have to experiment with a few methods and see what works best. But that's all part of the process. Generally speaking, you should start your meditation practice by sitting down for twenty or thirty minutes only once or twice a week. This will ease you into the habit of meditating. Once you've established the habit, however, you can increase your meditation practices to once a day for however long you find helpful.

It is also important to note that your meditation style may change over time. You may also find that your mood, location, or physical health affects the manner of meditation you prefer. This is completely normal. As with all things in meditation, learning to listen to your body or mind and follow its cues is part of your practice.

Guided Meditation Exercises

Now that you know the types of meditation you can choose from, it is time to begin your meditation practice. The rest of this chapter is dedicated to a few guided meditations to start you off. You can use these for as long as you like, though you may find yourself developing your own meditation path or looking up new ones when you've memorized the ones in this book.

The guided meditations in this book – as well as most you'll find in other sources – are written based on the traditional model of meditating. You are free to adapt them for your practice, however. Add ambient sound or a visual focus if it suits you. If you prefer moving meditation, ignore instructions to sit or lie down. The meditations below are intended to act as strong frames on which you can build your own meditation practice.

Your first guided meditation will teach you how to center. This is a method through which you acknowledge all the directions in which you're being pulled, then find your balance between them all. The second meditation will help you ground yourself within that center point. And, finally, the third meditation is a basic guide on learning to let your thoughts come and go without latching onto them as you meditate.

This third meditation practice is the one you're most like to perform throughout the day as you become more accustomed to it. Once you get the hang of it, you'll find yourself practicing short bursts of meditation between meetings at work, as you work on housework, or when you're out with friends and overwhelmed. It is a handy tool that you can use to find a bit of calm anywhere you are. Grounding and centering, on the other hand, are best practiced either in the morning or at night. Or, if you're particularly busy, they can help renew your focus before an event, meeting, or presentation.

Basic Centering

Before you begin meditating, find a quiet place that suits your needs. If you have chosen moving meditation, you will also want to ensure that you won't bump into or trip over anything. Likewise, you'll want to find a place with decent ventilation if you plan on lighting candles of incense. Smoke can be excellent for visual meditation. But it is very unpleasant to breathe when it builds up.

When you have found a good space, make sure you won't be disturbed. Set your phone to silent or shut it off, if you can. Let anyone else in your household know that you need some time to yourself. And, if necessary, you may want to lock the door to the room where you're meditating. This might seem extreme. But, until you are more experienced, it will be very easy for you to lose your concentration.

You may also want to bring a notebook and a pen in the room with you. Although the point of this exercise is to center yourself at the hub of your energy, you may find that doing so inspires a number of thoughts. Part of the exercise is naming and grouping all the directions your energy goes. As you do this, you might find new ways to reduce your stress level or workload. You may also find commitments you can cut out or think of things you can change to improve how you spend your energy. If this happens, it's better to have a pen and paper nearby.

Now find a comfortable position. If you're using ambient noise, you'll want to make sure your headphones or earbuds won't become dislodged. Should you have a candle or stick of incense with you, you'll want to place this on a stable surface and find a seat close enough to watch the smoke or flame, while remaining far enough away that you won't inhale anything unpleasant.

To begin your meditation, close your eyes. Take as deep a breath as you can, counting the seconds it takes you to inhale fully. Hold your breath for two seconds. Now exhale and try to draw out your exhale until you count three more seconds for your exhale than your inhale.

Repeat this pattern until you feel yourself relaxing into the breath. You will feel some tension leave your shoulders, your hands may unclench or relax, and you may find that you can take deeper breaths as you go.

When this breathing pattern feels almost natural, begin thinking through all the commitments you have. If this causes stress, return your thoughts to your breathing until the tension fades back to its previous level. Then continue internally listing all the directions your energy must go.

With each direction you name, imagine a cord running from your core out toward the thing you're giving energy to. This could be a work commitment, a hobby, a person, or an illness you must manage. If you have to give energy to it, add it to your list.

Most people will feel a bit like a porcupine when they are in the midst of this meditation. Their energy will be going in every direction and, in their minds, they look like they're covered in spines. This is a representation of the stress that we carry in modern life. We have commitments that pull us in conflicting directions and rarely do we feel like there is enough energy for everything. And that is why centering is so important. From here – from this position of acknowledging your commitments – you're going to begin controlling them.

The next step – and the first step in controlling where your energy goes – is to collect each type of commitment. In your mind, assign a color to each type of commitment. Your specific categories may vary, but the most common are "work", "hobby", "romantic connections", "friendships", "family", and "health as you assign colors to your commitments, begin grouping them together.

Through all of this, try to maintain that deep, even breathing. If you find your breathing has become shallow or is speeding up, leave off with grouping your commitments and focus once again on your breathing until you're breathing deeply once more. Repeat this pattern as often as you need to until your commitments are grouped and your breathing remains deep.

Now, look at your commitments. Are there any you don't need and can cut out? If so, make a mental note to cut ties with those commitments as soon as you are done meditating. If you do choose to cut down on your commitments, make sure you're not cutting hobbies or other forms of self-care to make room for commitments to other people. If you don't take care of yourself, fulfilling other commitments will be much harder.

At this point, with your commitments under control and your breathing deep, imagine yourself taking all of your commitment in hand. Gather them up from where they radiate out from your body and hold them like reigns or balloon ribbons in one hand. As you do this, think to yourself that you are taking control of how much energy goes to each thing. Your commitments can no longer draw energy from you whenever they want. You must allow them access before they can tap into your personal energy. In this way, you are centered as the guardian of your energy.

Open your eyes or shift them away from your visual focus. If you chose to cut down on your commitments, write down which you chose to cut and the steps you must take to do so. Next, write down any other thoughts you have about how you spend your energy. Did you think of ways to reduce your workload? Are there areas where you need more energy coming in? Can you combine commitments to reduce your stress level? Write down your thoughts and keep them in a safe place. You may find yourself returning to them as you work through the changes you want to make in your life.

Basic Grounding

Grounding and centering often go together. You do not have to do them one right after the other, however. You might find it helpful to center in the morning, so you approach your day in control of your energy, and then ground at night. Grounding, generally, helps you find or return to your bedrock, your foundation. By grounding at the end of the day, you're letting go of any stress you might have picked up over the last few hours and preparing yourself for a calmer evening.

To ground, find a comfortable and secure place like you did when you centered. Follow the same steps to ensure you won't be bothered. And, as with centering, bring a notebook in case your practice shakes any thoughts lose that you want to remember. And, as with centering, make sure your space fits the type of grounding you want to do.

It will be a little more difficult to ground when moving, if only because of the visualization used in grounding meditations. You may find that you have to keep your feet in one place while moving the rest of your body, like a tree blowing in the wind. If this does not, you can try sitting and just moving your upper body.

When you're ready to begin your meditation, find a comfortable space and settle yourself. Use the same breathing practice as described in the centering exercise and focus on just your breathing until the slow, deep pace of it feels natural. When you have achieved this, turn your attention to the way the ground feels beneath you.

Feel the way that the ground supports you and make a note of everywhere you can feel your body touching the floor. If any negative self-talk starts at this phase, pause and actively counsel yourself into a more compassionate inner monologue. Then return your attention to the ways your body is connected to the ground.

Carry this sensation of support with you as you visualize yourself in your mind. Imagine that same feeling of support providing a foundation for your inner self. Let that sense of security support your thoughts, your feelings, and your sense of confidence in yourself. Take a moment to appreciate that you are doing this for yourself, that you are providing yourself with a sense of support and stability.

Now call to mind all the times you felt out of step throughout the day. This could be a time when someone upset you or when you were abruptly reminded of something you forgot. Let yourself remember any time when you felt as though your foundation were not as stable as it is at this very moment. You might have to pause between recollections and return your focus to your breathing. This is perfectly normal and part of giving your inner monologue some order.

When you have gone over your day, hold these memories in your mind and then tell yourself that these things happen. That you sometimes get thrown off your rhythm and you lose touch with your foundation. But here, at the end of the day, you're back on your foundation. None of those moments created a permanent, lasting negative effect. If you worry, they may cause future negative effects, remind yourself that you can always come back to your foundation. That your foundation is something you can never truly lose.

With this affirmation in mind, open your eyes and go about the rest of your day. If you've chosen to do this right before bed, go through your nighttime routine and keep the affirmation in mind as you fall asleep. You can also use this affirmation as a touchstone through the following day whenever you next feel that you're losing touch with your foundation.

Letting Go of Your Thoughts

Although this exercise might seem like the first thing you should learn when you meditate, it's actually the perfect follow-up to grounding and centering. Both grounding and centering encourage you to call upon specific thoughts and memories, which allows your mind to latch onto them the way it normally would. Letting go of your thoughts, however, requires your mind to become more passive with its own thoughts. And that is harder than it sounds.

Many people have the idea that meditation requires you to completely empty your mind of all thoughts. And while some people can do this, most people cannot. This is why many meditation teachers now instruct their students to become more passive with their thoughts. When you are passive with your thoughts, you can let your mind stay as busy as it always it. You simply hold a simpler focus and let your unconscious mind process all the things your conscious mind is usually preoccupied with.

For the purpose of this exercise, your focus will be your breathing. At some point, you may choose to create a mental construct that will hold your attention. But, for now, you're going to build on the breathing practice you started with your grounding and centering meditations.

Maintaining your focus on your breathing is absolutely key for this type of meditation. The instructions are deceptively simple. But it will practice before you are able to let your thoughts come and go without paying them too much attention.

Prepare yourself as you did with your other meditations. Find a location well-suited to your type of meditation and get settled. Start counting your breathing by taking as deep a breath as possible. Hold this breath for two seconds, then slowly let it out. Try to take three seconds longer to exhale than you did to inhale. Pause one second then repeat this process.

As you focus on your breathing, your mind will continue producing thoughts like it always does. When a thought tries to intrude on your breathing, gently remind yourself that you're thinking about your breathing right now. Then actively return to counting your breaths.

You may find that your breathing gets deeper as you continue to meditate. You might also find yourself become emotional as you let your thoughts roam where they please. This is just your subconscious mind processing your thoughts for you. Acknowledge the feelings and accept that they are normal and acceptable. But try your best to keep your focus on your breathing.

When you first begin using this meditation, you should aim to do it for five minutes. You can set a timer or ask someone to come get you when the five minutes are up. As you become more experienced, increase this time until you're up at twenty to thirty minutes at a time. Some people find that they enjoy their meditations and want to extend their time even further. Others limit their deep meditations to a few times a week and simply use the breath counting to aid their calm through the week. Do whatever works for you.

A Final Note

Meditation might not have been a part of your life before you picked up this book. But that doesn't mean you can't find utility in it. For some people, it is a spiritual practice. For others, it is a way to get a better handle on their energy and their thoughts. In both cases, it creates a stronger connection between your mind and your body.

This connection will let you check in with yourself more regularly. And while this might not seem like something you need to consciously do, think about how often you over-extend yourself. Everyone has committed to too many things, given ground on their emotional boundaries, or worked too hard at the gym. Meditation might not help you avoid these situations entirely. But being more in touch with both your own body and your own mind can help you reduce how often these things happen.

Listening to your comfort cues, both mental and physical, is key for a long and healthy life. Anyone with a sports injury or who has had to extract themselves from a toxic situation will attest to this. It is best to avoid the situation entirely than have to cope with the fallout after the fact. So, stay checked in with yourself. And keep these skills fresh as you move on to the other changes waiting on your journey.

CHAPTER 2

EDUCATION

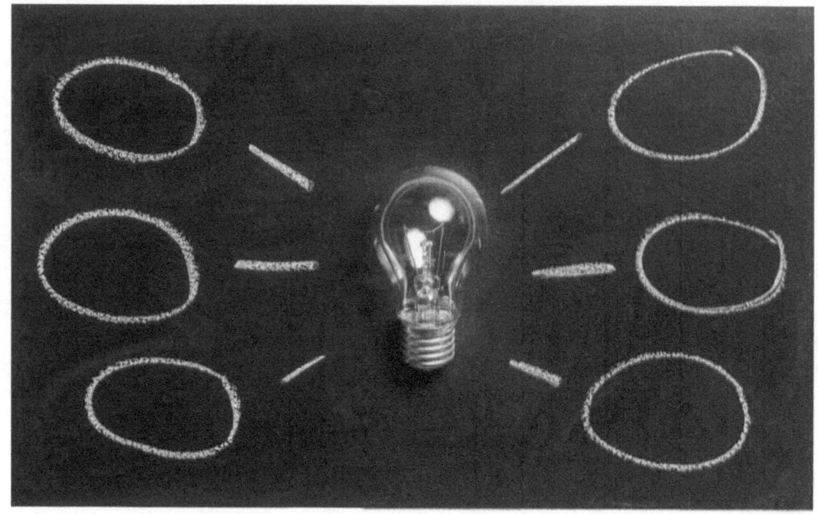

Learning to control your energy, talk to yourself with compassion, and let your thoughts flow freely are all hallmarks of a healthy internal life. And while these skills are important, they must be paired with healthy mental stimulation.

No matter which direction you want to take your life, you're going to have to learn something. It might be a new skill, new social cues, hiking trails. Every change requires that we learn something new. This chapter will help you find the best ways to learn the new information you need to know. It will cover the difference between education and learning as well as several different methods for getting the information you need.

The Power of Learning

Our brains crave stimulation. Logic puzzles, crosswords, and other brain teasers have long been recommended as ways for people to keep their minds sharp as they age. And anyone with children will tell you that letting them learn a new skill is a good way to keep them preoccupied for a good, long while.

But learning does even more. Learning new skills opens up new channels of communication and new avenues of social connections. Depending on how you learn your new skills or information, you're putting yourself in a position to make friends with people who share your interests. And, depending on the information or skill you're learning, you might be able to exercise your body at the same time you're stimulating your mind.

New skills and new information also stimulate the creative centers of our brain. Creativity happens when our minds take different pieces of information and combine them in new and novel ways. We do this because our brain craves novelty. Lucky for us, the end result is usually amusing and sometimes, if we're lucky, a little bit awe-inspiring.

And sometimes, if we're lucky, learning something new can give us new energy in our lives. Artists and writers around the world have said time and again that honing their creative skills gave them new vigor for life. People in a variety of fields have told the story of finding their calling and finally feeling a sense of purpose. And, when people are particularly down, learning new skills may give them something to look forward to in order to raise their spirits.

Learning truly is one of the greatest gifts humanity has given itself. And just as learning has a variety of benefits, there are a variety of ways you can learn. But before we dive into those, I want to touch on the difference between learning and education.

Education Versus Learning

Everyone knows someone who hated school. You might even be that person. But when most people talk about what they hated in school, it wasn't the information they were given. It was how the information was presented. The teacher was boring or the tests were confusing. Math is a mystery and none of it applies to real-life anyway!

These complaints have been around, literally, since some of humanity's earliest written records. Students have always complained about how their information was presented and teachers have always complained that their students aren't paying attention. It's a cycle that humanity has yet to break.

But there does seem to be hope. Many people now acknowledge that information might have to be presented a few times in different ways before everyone can get it. And, in cases like math, shifting the focus from "find the right answer" to "this is how the process works" is an important distinction we need to make.

So, what does all of this mean for you as you're making changes in your life? Well, given that you're probably an adult who has already gone through a fair amount of formal education, it means you decide how you're going to learn the information you seek.

If lectures could never hold your attention, reading at your own pace in an online class might be better. And if you had trouble sitting still during class, you might now do better with an audiobook playing while you go for a run. You already know what you don't like when you're being educated. Now you get to find the things you do like.

Education is the process through which you learn. Learning is simply the act of gathering and processing information. So, if you don't thrive in one educational model, you now have the power to try out another. And if that one doesn't work for you, try yet another. You're on a journey to change the direction of your life which means you need to find the things that work best for you. And, as we talked about in chapter one, you need to show yourself compassion as you search for your ideal educational style.

Finding Your Education Path

Not that long ago, learning a new skill meant going to a formal school and attending classes. This might have been a university or a trade school. But no matter the establishment, you still worked under a single teacher and were limited by the options offered through the school you attended.

If you're planning to make a career out of the new things you learn, this is still the best option. Especially if you're learning a trade. But if you're learning a new skill or exploring a new topic solely for your own enjoyment – or for gains outside of a formal career – you now have a wide range of ways you can choose to learn.

You might still find a traditional establishment the most appealing option. With formal schools, you can be certain the teachers have been tested and know their stuff. You can also trust that they're getting their information from reputable sources so that you, in turn, have accurate information. But these schools are often expensive and very rigid in their timing and teaching styles.

This is where alternatives come in handy. You might find an online course that better suits your needs. If you choose to attend an online school, make sure to check their accreditation and reputation beforehand. Once that checks out, you may find a wider range of classes and the ability to learn on your own schedule.

There are also fewer formal options available. Online courses abound for all sorts of things from plumbing to sewing to mythology to storytelling. Your local library might even offer access to online classes through the use of your library card. They are literally that common. You do, however, run the risk of getting a teacher who doesn't know their content quite as well. Or they might be excellent teachers who found a bad source without realizing it. When learning in this format, it's always a good idea to use your discretion and look up anything that seems off.

And there are yet more options. Some community centers offer life skills classes that range from cooking to sewing to basic tax preparation. And if you want to learn a crafty skill – anything from makeup application to cooking to car repair – there are plenty of videos online. The creators know their stuff, they just don't have the same professional placement as a professor. Online videos, in particular, are a great way to dip your toes into a subject before you dive in with pricier classes.

You can follow one avenue of learning or you can mix and match approaches. In addition to all of these options, there is always self-guided learning. Once you find your passion, you'll likely end up adding this approach to your learning toolbox whether or not you realize it at first. Self-guided learning usually takes the form of reading up on a topic and simply following your interests as you find new information that catches your eye.

The Social Side of Learning

When you were younger, you probably made most of your friends in the schoolyard. And, as you got older, your friends changed, depending on who you spent the most time with while in school. Friendships formed during our school years sometimes last the rest of our lives.

But, once we graduate from school, it suddenly becomes difficult to make friends. Some people rely on their place of worship. Others might meet friends through school. And a local bar or pub has long been a gathering spot for adults. But what if you don't drink or don't have a place of worship? And despite the importance of work friends, it can be hard to transition from work friends to friends in your off-hours.

Exploring a new topic or hobby opens up so many ways to meet people. At a base level, your studies will probably get you out of the house. Even online courses usually urge you to go out and buy new books or explore certain kinds of locations or people watch. You can also find online groups that give you a chance to meet other people in your community that share your interests.

If your educational path takes you outside your home, the options are even more pronounced. Trade schools and universities create a space where students can mingle before and after class. Many schools also offer student groups as well that cater to both casual and professional interests.

Unlike work friends, you will share a strong positive connection with people you meet while pursuing your interests and passions. Friendships are easier to create and maintain if you can share something more than workplace gossip and opinions on the latest office policy. And, as you pursue your interests, your new friends will be just as interested in your newest discoveries as you are!

Finding Your Passion

If you're reading this chapter, you want to add more learning into your life. People who want to focus on learning usually fall into one of two categories: people want to learn everything and don't know where to start, or people who have the urge to learn but don't know what specific direction to go. Neither situation is helpful. And both can leave you feeling so frustrated you're not sure how to move forward. In this section, I will suggest a writing exercise for both situations so that you can use the one that best suits your needs.

So Much to Learn, So Little Time

People with a love of learning often run into this problem. They have so much they want to learn that they can't choose which topic, to begin with. If you're one of these people, you have my sympathies. I have been in your shoes. The writing exercise in this section will help you narrow down your interests and put them into a prioritized list.

You're going to need quite a bit of paper for this exercise. Blank paper will work best. You will also want a pen or pencil as well as either an extensive set of highlighters, markers, or colored pencils. As with the meditation chapter, you'll want to make sure you can run through this exercise at least once without being disturbed. The space doesn't need to be quite as secure, but you will want to let people know that you need time to work without any interruptions.

Make sure you're seated somewhere you will be comfortable, even if you're sitting for an extended period of time. To begin, just keep your pen and paper in front of you. The highlighters, markers, or colored pencils are for a color-coding process that will not come into play right away. And if you try to color-code as you go, you will very likely get sidetracked.

This writing exercise will use a thought web to help you narrow down which interests tend to weigh on your thoughts most heavily. Not only that, but it will help you break down that interest into subcategories that may be more in line with the specific interest you have.

At first glance, this might seem like overkill, but it can help if you're feeling overwhelmed. If, for example, you want to get into hand lettering, you might be intimidated by the sheer amount of information. But as you work on your idea web you might find that you're actually interested in hand-lettering chalkboard signs. So instead of learning about ink pens and oil crayons and how to measure your lettering on heavy paper, you can focus on learning skills associated with chalk and chalkboards.

Achieving this kind of focus is easy when you break your thoughts down into a web. It's a simple and intuitive process, but it can be time-consuming and – if you have a *lot* of interests – it can take up a fair amount of paper.

The first step is to take a few deep breaths and push aside other thoughts. If you've already gone through the meditation chapter, this is a good time to do a quick run-through of the centering exercise. You don't want to ignore all of your thoughts, of course. But you will want to set aside thoughts that aren't related to your current project. Forget about bills that you have to pay or social engagements that are coming up. This might relate to your interests but those actions themselves are not part of your focus right now.

With your mind focused on exploring your interests, write down the first thing that comes to your mind. Write it in the center of the page and draw a circle around it. If your thoughts are stuck on this interest, go ahead and start drawing lines that branch off the main bubble. Write down each thought at the end of its own branch, then circle it like you circled the original idea. Keep adding new ideas to the main bubble or start branching off the secondary ideas. You can add as many layers of branches as you want. And each layer can hold as many ideas as you want. Later you'll have to pare these back or combine them. But, for now, just go where your mind takes you and write down everything it comes up with.

If you come up with one main topic and then come up with a new topic, grab a new sheet of paper. Each idea should have its own page so that you have plenty of room to build on each main interest. Use as many sheets of paper as you need. And, in case you want to come back to these ideas later on and take on another new topic, you might want to keep these pages in their own folder or binder when you're done.

As you go, you may find that you come up with one or two main ideas and then jump back to a more detailed interest related to the main idea you wrote down before. Go back and add it in! There is no rule saying you only have to work on the most recent idea you wrote down.

You might also come up with a secondary idea that belongs to more than one main idea. If, for example, you want to learn more about dance and a particular part of your heritage, a subtopic that comes up might be a traditional dance from that particular part of your family tree. It is acceptable – encouraged, even – for you two write this more detailed interest down under both main ideas. Later, when you're color-coding, you can put a special symbol next to this idea so that you can see, at a glance, how it connects more than one of your main interests.

Keep going until you've run out of interest. This might happen in a few minutes or you might look up to see that you've been brainstorming for an hour or more. There is no wrong time to stop. Just go for as long as your mind wants to toss out ideas.

When your mind quiets down, set down your pen and shake out your fingers. Get up and stretch your legs, or get a glass of water. Look at something other than your idea webs for a few minutes so that you can come back to them with fresher eyes. When you're feeling rested after mining your ideas, return to your idea webs.

This is where your markers, highlighters, or colored pencils will come in handy. Look at each idea in turn. Just as you grouped your commitments into color-coded bundles when you did your centering meditation, you are going to group your ideas into general categories. Are some academic in nature? Do you see a lot of arts and crafts skills in your webs? Have you found yourself preoccupied with practical skills like auto repair, home improvement, or gardening? Or, perhaps, are you more interested in the physical side of learning?

As you sort your ideas into groups, assign each group a color. Now, go through the ideas that branch out from your main interests. If any of the smaller ideas fall into a different category as their parent idea, color code them to match the category they do belong to. When you've gone through everything, set aside your markers and look at which color appears most often.

This color-coding system will help guide you as you begin to explore your interests. You should start with the interest type that appears most often. You are already giving so much of your mental energy to the topic that it makes sense for your physical energy to go into it as well.

You can also use these color-coded webs to create action plans. If you want to learn how to create printable planner pages, for example, you know you'll have to learn the ins and outs of design software, the size of most planners, and how to operate any printers or sticker cutters you'll have to use.

Your color-coding system can also help if you are the type to use a planner or calendar. You can write lessons related to your passion in a color that matches your color web. Should your interest require study materials, you can match your notebooks and pens to the color you assigned on your web. This does more than create a sense of aesthetic symmetry. It creates a link between that color, your materials, and the topic that inspired you in the first place. Every time you look at your study supplies or an entry on your calendar for an event related to your interest, you'll be reminded of why you started your journey in the first place.

Putting a Pin in Your Passion

Sometimes we get the urge to learn something new, but we have no idea what direction to go. We know that we're restless for mental stimulation. But there just isn't one specific thing that jumps to mind when we're trying to pick a topic. If this sounds like you, don't despair. There is hope!

In books and movies, finding your passion usually requires some grand adventure. The protagonists in these tales take off and jet around the world or give up everything to find out what really drives them. This is a grand, romantic notion that might appeal to you. And, if it does, don't let me stop you!

But if you're not looking to spend your life – or if jetting around the world is a bit beyond your means – there are other options. With a little bit of visualization, some dedicated time to concentrate, a pen, and some paper, you can at least give yourself a foothold in finding your passion.

Of course, you can always dive into learning without a direction. Most college students have known at least one person who just takes any class that sounds remotely interesting until they find something that really hooks their interest. There is absolutely nothing wrong with this method. Provided you can afford it, of course. On the off-chance that you're the type to crave a *little* more direction than that, I've come up with a writing exercise to help get your foot in the door before you even touch a course catalog or head to the local library.

To begin, gather up some paper, a pen, and one or two highlighters. Find a comfortable and private place to work, much like the place you found for your meditation practices in the last chapter. You don't need quite as much privacy because you won't be concentrating as hard. But you will want to let the people in your household know that you need to work without interruption. And it might be a good idea to leave your phone in another room or put it face-down at the other end of the table do you don't get distracted.

Once you're settled in a comfortable seat, close your eyes and imagine your ideal self. This can be the same ideal self as the one from your meditation practice. Or, if you want to focus more specifically on your interests, you can create an ideal self in a situation where you would be discussing your interests.

As you imagine this ideal self, begin writing down details that relate to something you would have to learn. Are you dressed in the latest fashion, which would require learning some design skills? Maybe you're hosting a dinner party that would require you to learn new culinary skills. Or perhaps your ideal self is spending time alone, painting or playing an instrument you have yet to try.

Write down each detail as you notice it. If one particular detail catches your eye, put a star next to it. You can even note details like the haircut or makeup your ideal self might be wearing. If you're not good at styling your own hair or you struggle to apply makeup, those could be new skills to try and learn. You don't have to stop at one visualization. You can create as many ideal forms of yourself as you'd like. Just write down the details of each one and try to use a separate sheet of paper for each ideal form.

When you're done, get up take a bit of a stroll. Shake out your fingers, get a glass of water, and generally spend some time thinking about something other than the lists you just made. This will let you come back to the project with a fresh set of eyes.

After you've had a chance to walk around for a bit, return to your seat in front of your lists. Pick up your highlighter and start reading over your lists. Every time you come across a detail that really catches your attention, highlight that sentence. If you see the same kind of detail popping up over and over, put a special symbol next to it. This way you can come back to those repeat details after you've got the through the list once.

Read through all the details you've written down, then go back to the ones you highlighted. Reread just those details and see if there is a common theme or even a couple of common themes. Write each theme in the center of its own sheet of paper and put a circle around it. This theme will form the basis for an idea web.

With a specific theme at the center of the page, your mind has something to focus on. You might not get any new ideas. But, as you look at the theme and read over the details that brought you to this point, you might realize that there is something specific you want to learn about that theme.

If you wrote down "cooking", for example, you probably don't want to learn everything there is to know about cooking. But if the detail that led you here was "hosting a dinner party where I served a roast chicken" and you don't know how to roast a chicken, you know you have a place to start.

Such a tiny detail might not seem that important. It's a roast chicken, after all. Or maybe it's an acoustic guitar, or learning to knit a scarf, or knowing a few words in a language your ancestors once spoke. Whatever the detail, remind yourself that small does not mean insignificant. Your mind took the time to furnish that small detail. It is something intensely personal, much like the changes you're making in your life to improve your odds of living longer and enjoying your time a little bit more.

Keep these small details close and use them as a reference point when you start making your action plans. Returning to the roast chicken example, you might need to check out a library book, buy a chicken, and then set aside some pizza money in case you don't get it right the first time. That would be your action plan. It doesn't have to be fancy or complicated. It just has to work for you.

You might find that the small detail you latched onto this time doesn't lead you very far down a path you find interesting. That is where all the other details come in handy. Or, conversely, you might find that learning that one small skill – or those few words, or that small bit of information – leads you into a realm of learning you never considered. What started as one roast chicken might lead to cooking your way through an interesting cookbook, recipe by recipe.

That's the beauty of learning. Even if you start with a tiny seed, it can take you to amazing places. You just have to be willing to explore.

A Final Note

Mental health has long been linked to maintaining our quality of life as we age. And stimulating your mind is a good way to keep it sharp. The best part is, you can start at any age and still reap the benefits as you get older.

You might choose to dig into a new branch of history you've never explored. Or you might decide that it's time to start a new hobby. Whatever your new interest, pursuing your passion can lead you to new places you never expected.

Perhaps you'll meet new friends. Or you might find that one passion leads to another and another until you're exploring whole new worlds. In some cases, your new interests might even branch into new ways to stay active. If this is the direction your interests go, check out the next chapter. It will help you maximize the benefits of your newfound passion.

CHAPTER 3

PHYSICAL ACTIVITY

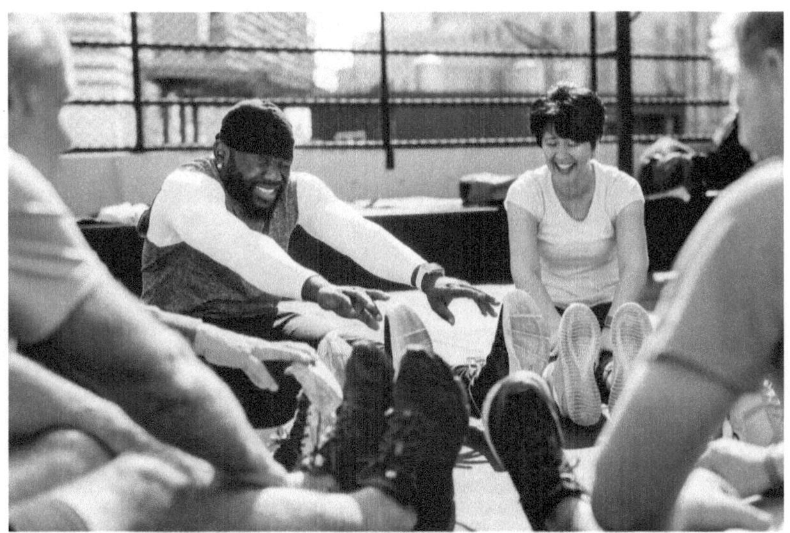

When we talk about extending our lifespans or improving our health, a lot of people immediately think about their weight. But getting active shouldn't revolve around the number on your scale. And that is why this chapter's scope goes much further than that. My goal is to make physical activity appealing and fun, even if you're not usually the "get up and go" type.

Physical activity keeps us flexible while stimulating both our muscular and skeletal systems. There is even mounting evidence that certain kinds of exercise can help maintain bone density as we age. On top of all that, physical exercise has also been linked to an improved sense of mental clarity. Together, all of this reminds us that our bodies and minds are interconnected. And that supporting one is a great way to support the other.

Since you're reading this chapter, I can safely assume that one of the changes you want to make in your life is to increase your physical activity. But as anyone who has tried to form a gym habit can tell you, physical activity is hard to get a taste for. Yes, some people take to it quickly. But, for most people, it takes a little trial and error to find out what sort of physical activity suits you best.

This chapter should help narrow down the search. It will cover the importance of physical activity beyond weight loss as well as how to connect the physical activity to other interests you might have. There will also be tips to help you get started, suggestions on taking things to the next level, and even some unique fitness suggestions that might be a little more fun than another trip to the gym.

More than Weight Loss

Physical fitness – for a lot of reasons – has become hyper-focused on the idea of weight loss. And that's not a good thing. Yes, some people want to get active so that they can lose weight. If this is the case for you, know there is absolutely nothing wrong with making that choice for yourself. But if, on the other hand, you're not interested in losing weight, there are still plenty of reasons to be active. Whichever way your interests lie, there is some kind of physical activity out there to fit your needs.

Getting active should be about the way it makes your body feel. At first, on the surface, you're probably going to feel sore and tired. These aren't fun sensations, but they are both temporary. More than that, they don't matter when compared to the sense of accomplishment you feel when you get to the other side of a tough goal. Or, if you're learning something new, the elation you feel when you're the one doing something you once thought was far beyond your skillset.

Moving your body also does all sorts of wonderful things for your health, both mental and physical. When you are in the habit of moving your body, you become much more aware of how it moves. This will help improve your balance, make you more aware of the space around you and how you move in it. In addition, it can help you avoid injury from strain or overuse.

Frequent motion also keeps you limber so that you're less likely to injure yourself. Many people also find that consistent physical activity helps them maintain a more positive or peaceful outlook while giving them an outlet for any restless energy they have.

Moving your body should be about showing yourself compassion. Chapter one covered compassionate self-talk and changing your inner monologue to be gentler on yourself. Building on that theme, this chapter aims to highlight the ways that physical activity is a gift you give yourself. Not a way to punish yourself for the food you eat or what you look like.

Changing your life for the better is not about making yourself suffer until you achieve a certain goal. It is about finding ways to be happy with the way you are while still pursuing your hopes and aspirations. Physical activity is part of that.

Finding the Connections

No matter what your passion is, you can add physical activity to the mix. Though each interest is different, there are a few key ways to involve a component that gets you up and moving. This section will outline a few of those methods and give examples. You might not see your exact interest among those outlined here. But I am confident that, using these tips, you can find a way to move your body and still pursue your interests.

Find a Theme

I know all interests run on a theme. But for this example, you'll need to focus on a smaller theme within your overall interest. If you're a chef, for example, you could find events themed on ending hunger. Or if your interest lies in painting, you could find events that honor famous painters or expose people to more art.

These events will usually be fundraising marathons and many of them welcome walkers, people on scooters, and even people pulling their children in wagons. Marathons aren't just the realm of avid runners anymore. With a little digging, you're sure to find an event that suits you.

If you're not looking for something quite that intense, you might find something like an art walk to be more your speed. These events encourage people to walk from one gallery to another – usually, galleries that are on a prescribed route and part of the event – or from one local shop to another so people can view work by local artists.

You might also find farmer's markets or swap meets well suited to your tastes. Both events fall into the scope of your theme (cooking for the first, art for the second) and both get you up and moving. The movement might not get your heart pounding or make you sweat. But it still gets you in motion and that's the most important thing.

Follow the History

A lot of interests are rooted in layers of rich history. This is especially true of interests like crafting, cooking, and most historical research. If your interests fall into any of these categories, you can probably find something related to the history of your topic that can get you on your feet.

Certain interests, like researching a culture or country your family is connected to, has lots of options. You can learn a dance from that culture. Or, if you can go to that location, you can arrange a walking tour of important sites.

Should your topic fall into a territory like crafting, on the other hand, you might have to get a little more creative. Let's take knitting as an example. Knitting is, for the most part, a stationary activity. It always has been and, unless you're on a stationary bicycle, it probably always will be. But that doesn't mean you should give up hope.

Many knitters develop an interest in where the fiber for their projects comes from. If you are one such knitter, you can probably find a sheep or alpaca farm that offers tours of their grounds. Many of these farms also have orchards, extended tours or "pick your own" crops that offer even more chances to keep your body moving while supporting people in your interest's community.

And you don't have to limit yourself to tours that other people offer. Sewers, for example, can look up locally-owned fabric or quilting shops and create a "tour" by visiting each one and spending some time perusing the shops. If you go this route, it is usually polite to at least buy something small from the shops you visit so that you're supporting them. As an added bonus, you may find that some of these shops offer classes of get-togethers that can either support you as you learn the skill or help you forge social connections.

Look for a Group

In the last section, I mentioned that touring locally owned shops might yield groups that connect people with shared interests. This is a great way to meet new people, but it might also be a fun way to incorporate your interests into everyday physical activity.

A lot of people enjoy going on a daily walk. It helps them clear their heads and gather their thoughts. Daily walks also provide a gentle and easily customizable way for people to work some motion into their daily lives. And while these can be fun, they would be even better if you shared them with people who had other interests in common with you.

If you already attend a crafting group, ask around to see if anyone would like to take your crafty conversations along for a walk. And, of course, this isn't just restricted to crafting. Ask classmates if they want to go over notes while you're walking around campus. Check out with people in your local meetup group to see if they want to go on a gentle hike through some nearby hills while you talk about whatever it is that connects you.

You might even find success with this by checking in with your gym to see if you can post fliers. There might be other people in your circles that would love to chat about any and every interest you're focused on while you rack up laps around the track or work up a sweat on the elliptical machine.

Go Meta

This tip is probably going to resonate a little more with the nerds among the readers than with others. But anyone can use it. By "go meta", I mean to look at the details of your interests and find something in those details that you then turn around and make active.

People with an interest in pop culture or history will both have an easy time of this. As an example, let's take people who are very into either Star Trek or the Regency era of British history. Star Trek fans can learn any one of the various fighting styles referenced in the franchise.

People with an interest in the Regency era can do something very similar. They can learn any one of the various past times enjoyed by people in that era, from horseback riding to sword fighting to dancing.

People in both groups could easily go online and find other people with similar interests that would happily learn these activities with them. And this is an absolutely fantastic opportunity to combine three ways in which you can both prolong your life and improve its quality. You will get your body moving while learning something new and forging social connections.

Although I focused on two very easy examples in this section, you can easily turn this tip onto nearly any topic. All you have to do is look at the information that surrounds or cushions your interest. Look at the time period in which it was set or when it was most popular. Do a little digging and see what sports or physical hobbies were also popular at the time.

Starting Off Easy

By now you probably have some idea of how you're going to get yourself moving. And there's a good chance you're even excited to get started, whether or not you're generally an active person. But before you dive in, you need to make sure you're not pushing yourself too hard.

I don't want to discourage anyone from trying new or difficult things. Quite the opposite, actually. But as you're diving into your new activity, make sure you're listening to your body's cues. If you feel your muscles straining to a painful degree or if your chest feels so tight, you're struggling to breathe, take a break.

Our bodies send us these signals for a reason. Ignoring warning signs can lead to injury or worse if you're not careful. And this is especially true if you haven't been generally active in the past. No matter how fun the activity is or how excited you are, it is always best to start slow.

The best way to do this is to limit the time you spend on your activity. If you're a generally active person, you can probably handle putting yourself through your paces a few times a week.

But if you're someone who generally lives a more sedentary lifestyle, you might want to start off with only one or two days of activity a week. And, on those days, you should probably limit yourself to twenty or thirty minutes. If the activity isn't one that's meant to make you sweat or get your heart racing, you might be able to go for an hour on your active days.

Starting off slow is not a bad thing. By giving yourself time to learn your body's cues, you're improving your chances of making physical activity a more common habit. Starting slowly also gives you a good baseline for what you can handle before you add in more activity. And, if you keep a log of your activity levels, you can look back and see your progress as you go along.

Taking Things to the Next Level

There are a few ways you can bump up your activity level when you're ready. The easiest options are to either increase the amount of time you spend moving on your active days, or to increase how many days a week you're active.

Both of these options give you a lot of flexibility in how exactly you increase your activity levels. If you decide to increase how long you're active on certain days, you can increase the time by as little as ten minutes or as much as an hour. The new duration depends on your comfort level, that's it.

Adding more active days, on the other hand, could be as simple as going for a few more walks each week. But if your active option requires a group or a class, you might find it a little more difficult to increase the number of days you're up and moving.

If you run into a snag like this, there's nothing stopping you from adding a new kind of activity. If you picked up a form of dance or martial arts, for example, you can practice your form on your days off. Or, if that is unappealing, you could start a yoga practice to improve your flexibility and breathing.

People who need to add more active days to their week might also want to consider investing in simple home workout equipment. Light hand weights – between three and ten pounds each – are usually easy to find and affordable. Adding in new physical activity can be as simple as doing curls or overhead press exercises when a commercial comes on or while you're waiting for water to boil when you're cooking dinner.

Adding more activity to your day is easy. And, in many cases, it can even be fun. All it takes is a little innovation and the willingness to invest in yourself. You might think it's silly to lift weights while you're boiling water for dinner. But when those ten-pound weights go from annoyingly heavy to light as a feather, it will be a reminder that you built up your own strength just by taking things, gently, to the next level.

Unique Fitness Fun

So far, most of the suggestions in this chapter have been for fairly common forms of physical activity. Go for walks, try a marathon, take up dance, or try lifting weights when your arms are otherwise unoccupied at home. And, for many people, these suggestions are more than enough.

There are, however, people who need a little bit more depth to their activities. That is not to say that other activities aren't interesting. Some people just need a little something extra. For these people, they usually need an element of storytelling. Luckily, there are many options available that offer just such an experience.

Instead of just going for a walk at your local park, you can try walking around the nearest Renaissance fair when it opens. You can go in costume or in your street clothes, whatever is most comfortable for you. Or, if you don't have such an event opening up nearby any time soon, you can try to find a group of locals that incorporate role play into things like hiking, fencing, and other activities. This might seem far-fetched. But it's a much more common hobby than you would think.

There are also countless apps and programs that track your steps, then use these to reward you with in-game points and bonuses. Some of these games might be based on well-known franchises. Others are likely to be from independent developers and may offer a wide range of themes and storylines. If you don't know of any, just do a quick internet search for games or apps to use while working out. You will probably be surprised by the number of results you turn up.

And there are still more options. You can find a marathon, as mentioned earlier, that involves some sort of fantasy aspect. When zombies were a popular motif, there were plenty of events where people dressed up as the undead and walked for miles. There is no telling what might be available right this moment!

You can also try more niche activities, like paintball or laser tag. Far from being for children, these games are experiencing a resurgence as more people find that mixing fun and fitness yields amazing results. Games like Twister or tag also have adult variations that make them not only more difficult but more fun as well.

If you've read this far and still haven't found an activity to suit your needs, there is nothing stopping you from creating your own approach and inviting others to join! Several websites allow people to form groups where other locals can sign up to join you for nearly any interest. And, if you're interested, there's a good chance other people are too! You aren't limited to what other people can come up with. And, who knows? Maybe your custom-made method to get yourself active will become the next big thing and help others get up and get going.

A Final Note

Fitness, in all of its forms, should be about compassion. It isn't a means of punishing yourself for not measuring up to some social ideal. Rather, it's a way for you to give your body what it needs. And, done right, it can nourish your mind just as much as it supports your body.

Don't be afraid to mix and match different activity types. And be honest with yourself when something isn't working. Just because something is all the rage, or it worked before, does not mean that it is a viable option in your present.

As you begin adding more physical activity to your life, remember some of your lessons from chapter one. Be honest with yourself by acknowledging where you're really starting from and where you want to go. Don't let other people guide the changes you want to make in your life. This is your journey, these are your challenges. Only you get to decide how you approach them.

Even if you've never been big on physical fitness, the way you start moving your body now should be something fun. Dance lessons or strolling through a Renaissance fair every weekend might be out of the question. But you can still find ways to enjoy the ways you get yourself up and moving. And, yes, you might find yourself sore. But there's nothing wrong with that. Once the discomfort fades, you'll find that you can go just a little bit further and handle just a little bit more than you could before. And that is always a fantastic feeling.

CHAPTER 4
DIET AND NUTRITION

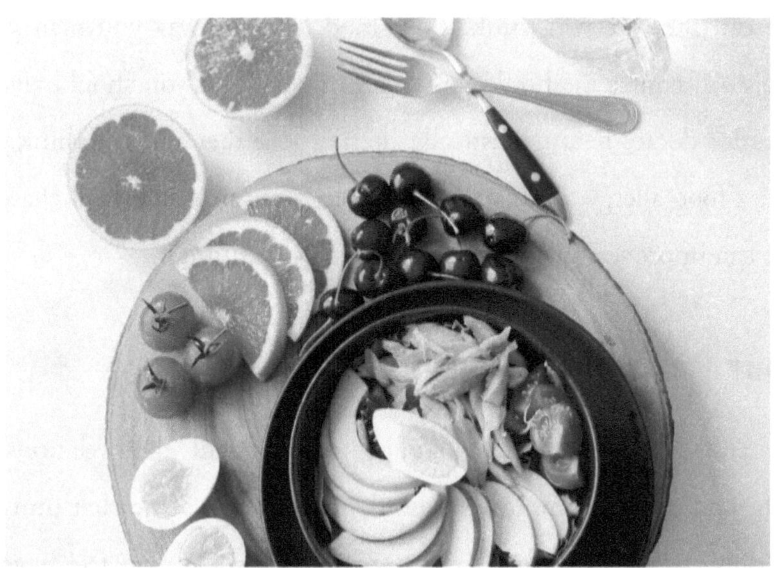

Food can be one of life's greatest joys. Unfortunately, it can also be the cause of – accidental and otherwise – a great deal of stress. Many people don't know what a good relationship with food looks like. They either fear gaining weight, don't know how to cook, or have a bad reaction to certain food with no idea how to track the cause.

But food doesn't have to be stressful. If you have a difficult relationship with food, you can change it. If you think you have a food allergy or sensitivity, there are ways to track your symptoms and pinpoint the cause. And if you're tired of the same old thing every week, there are easy ways to dive into new foods and new flavors.

This chapter will touch a little bit on every one of those topics. By the end of this chapter, you will have a solid basis for changing the way you eat, the way you think about food, and the way you plan your meals. Of course, it should go without saying that you should always consult a doctor before drastically altering your diet or if you think you have a food allergy. Until then, however, you can make small changes that can improve your life and the way food fits into it.

Your Relationship with Food

You've probably heard a lot of people talk about "their relationship with food". It's a common phrase that, despite its somewhat unusual wording, simply refers to the way food makes a person feel beyond "hungry" or "not hungry". Even if you think you don't have a relationship with food, there are probably certain dishes and flavors that pop to mind when you think of comfort. You have a positive relationship with those foods and flavors.

There are also, unfortunately, ways that you can have a bad relationship with food. If food is your only comfort, for instance, you might overeat. Or if you have been derided for your weight, all food regardless of type or flavor might cause feelings of guilt and anxiety.

Neither situation is ideal. And, in extreme cases, these negative feels toward food can lead to serious mental health issues.

If you're already suffering from such an issue, particularly if it takes the form of an eating disorder, please contact a hotline or hospital for help. It is admirable to take control of your mental health. But this book is not written to address the best way for you to do so. And you deserve the best help possible.

The tips in this section are intended for people who know they have a negative relationship with food but are not yet at the level where they need to seek outside help. Such a relationship might include general negative feelings toward food, including skipping a meal here or there just to avoid the strain of planning it out. Or it could include eating foods that you know upset your stomach but you're not sure how to cut from your diet.

I used to have this kind of relationship with food. If there wasn't anything pre-made in the fridge, like leftovers or a snack from the store, I would often skip lunch and just wait for dinner. This was an adult when I should have been able to prepare my own food. But the strain of choosing good, healthy recipes that I could make for just one person was often too much.

Things only became more frustrating when I discovered a few food intolerances. I ultimately found a good method for dealing with these issues, which I will outline in the *Allergies and Sensitivities* section of this chapter. But, until then, I avoided making my own food because I knew that something was making me sick and I just didn't want to bother with the side effects.

This is not a healthy way to approach food. Our bodies crave nourishment because it is where we get our energy from. Have you ever wondered why you crave food late at night, right before you're supposed to be going to bed? It's because your body is telling you it needs energy, either from sleep or from food. It's the same reason you get hungry throughout the day: your body is running low on energy.

I would repeat this fact to myself whenever I started feeling sluggish in the middle of the day. It reminded me why I was reaching for an apple or some tuna salad instead of a soda or candy bar. My body needed energy to keep me going, which meant I needed to give it good fuel sources. Otherwise, I would just be running low again soon.

This reminder also helped me lose a lot of my anxiety around eating. My weight had always been a focal point for me. And, because of this, I found that eating would sometimes cause me a lot of anxiety. I worried that I would eat too much or eat the wrong thing and gain more weight. But when I made that mental note about giving my body energy, I stopped worrying so much about the number on the scale. I changed my internal monologue from criticism to compassion, just as I outlined in chapter one. And, when I did, I found that I no longer feared my body's hunger signal. I welcomed it as a chance to take care of myself.

So, if you have these sorts of feelings toward food, write down this phrase: Food gives me the energy to pursue my goals. Food is showing my body compassion. Write it on the inside of your research notebooks, jot it down on a sticky note and attach it to your mirror. Scrawl it on a big sheet of construction paper and tape it to your fridge. Do whatever you have to do for the phrase to stick in your head.

Now every time you feel the negative feelings start to rise, close your eyes and repeat the phrase. Repeat as many times as you need before you can get yourself to prepare the food you know you should be eating. It might take time. And you might not manage it the first time you try it. But keep going and you will be able to slowly take control of your reactions.

You might wonder if this sort of stress is even worth it. And the answer is yes. I've already touched on the more severe mental health issues that can arise from negative connections to food. But there are less extreme – though still damaging – problems that can stem from thinking of food in a negative way.

At its least problematic, a negative relationship with food can turn every meal into a negative experience. Every time you crave food your mood will turn from good to bad to worse. That sort of stress isn't good for anyone. And this becomes a unique problem if your meals happen in groups. The groups could be friendly, professional, familial, or romantic. No matter the context, sitting down to every meal with a frown is bound to lead to conversations you don't want to have awkward meals that just reinforce your negative reaction.

There is no quick fix for negative thinking. Changing your relationship with food will take time and dedication. Above all, it will take believing in yourself. You might struggle with that at first. But, when you falter, return to the section on compassionate thinking in chapter one. Go through those tips again and then turn your attention back to your relationship with food.

These changes aren't easy but they are important. Living a long and healthy life requires that you stay in touch with both your body and your mind. Your relationship with food touches on both of these. Improving the way in which you interact with food lays a solid foundation for the next phase in changing the overall way food fits into your life: handling nutrition.

Nutrition's Wide Reach

You've heard of the food pyramid and the recommended five-a-day servings of fruits and vegetables. You might have even seen diagrams of dinner plates to show you how much of each thing you should be eating. Maybe you've heard of "first-sized servings" or the planning of your dinner based on ratios of vegetation to protein to carbs. We're bombarded all day every day with guidelines and rules on what, when, how, and where to eat.

But the truth of the matter is that nutrition is both more complex and simpler than putting five servings of vegetables on your plate every day or only eating the amount of meat you could fit in your palm at each meal. These were only ever meant to be basic guidelines but many people have become obsessed with following them almost to the letter. And it's getting in the way of how we all understand nutrition.

Rather than rely on the food pyramid, try looking at what kind of nutrients we need every day in order to keep our bodies healthy. Most governments have guidelines that break recommended serving sizes down into grams or other similar measurements. A quick internet search should turn up one for your area. If it doesn't, you can call your local doctor and ask if they have the link to the resource. Most offices will give it out even if you're not their patient.

Once you have the guidelines in hand, you'll want to look at where you can get the nutrients you need. Supplements are, of course, a perfectly acceptable option. But our bodies are better suited to absorbing nutrients from the food we eat. And you'll be surprised to see how many sources there are for all the nutrients on your newly-acquired list.

Let's take protein as the perfect example. For the most part, we only hear about animal-based protein sources. And this can be delicious. Chicken, milk, eggs, and cheese are all wonderful additions to just about any menu. But there are so many other protein sources you can choose from!

Most people can work with the animal-based sources. And, for the most part, many people *prefer* these sources. But there are a lot of reasons why someone might opt for plant-based sources. They might not want to eat animal products, they have food sensitivities, or they just don't like the taste. Whatever the reason, they have lots of options to choose from. From tempeh to spinach to mushrooms, the plant kingdom is full of protein options.

And this is just one example. As you look into the nutrients your body needs, you become more and more comfortable planning your own plate instead of relying on the diagrams or the food pyramid. And though this might be a little bit uncomfortable at first, it is ultimately a good thing. Because nutrition affects so much more than your waistline or how your plate is set up.

The nutrients we eat make their way into our very bones. They affect how our nails and hair grow. Our skin becomes dull when we don't get enough nutrients. And we feel energized when we get the doses we need. Meeting our nutrition requirements has been linked to a reduction in depression symptoms, bone density loss, and several negative effects of aging.

Understanding proper nutrition also takes some of the strain out of eating. When you know you need a certain amount of protein – not just a certain amount of meat – it becomes easier to work around restrictions like a need to cut back on fat or salt. You also feel a deeper connection with your body when you understand what it needs. It's not just a form that carries your mind around. Instead, it is part of you, a part that you understand the proper care and keeping of.

Proper nutrition will keep your body strong. And understanding what proper nutrition actually means will give you a stronger sense of connection to and control over your body. Instead of wondering if you've got the ratios right on your plate, you can focus on finding nutrient sources that taste good. It reduces stress and makes meals that much more enjoyable.

Allergies and Sensitivities

Allergies and sensitivities are another good reason for you to look into as many nutrient sources as possible. Avoiding foods, you react poorly to is much easier when you know of several alternatives that can fill the gap left behind. Of course, before you get to that stage, you have to pinpoint which foods are causing the negative reaction.

There are a few common signs and symptoms to look for if you think you might have a food allergy or sensitivity. The most obvious of this is a histamine or anaphylactic response. Both terms refer to a severe type of allergic reaction. Though some symptoms are very subtle, others are easy to spot. Hives, rashes, and facial swelling are all signs of an allergic response to a food.

If you have even a mild case of these reactions after eating a certain food, see a doctor right away. Mild reactions can get worse. And severe reactions can be life-threatening.

Although these symptoms are the most obvious – and the most dangerous – there are other symptoms you can look for. Symptoms like an upset stomach, gas, or frequent trips to the bathroom after certain foods may all point at a sensitivity. Food sensitivities are not quite as severe as allergies. In most cases, the person can still eat the food in question. But they suffer unpleasant side effects that, ultimately, might not be worth putting up with.

Other sensitivity symptoms include migraines, cottonmouth, and a marked increase in the intensity of mental health symptoms. People with anxiety will feel the effects more acutely and people with depression may find it harder to regulate their moods. Anyone with conditions will tell you that willingly dealing with symptom triggers is less than ideal.

But how are you supposed to identify which food – or compound in a food – is the culprit? The simple answer is that you use a food tracker tailored to the symptoms you have experienced. And this might sound complex or overwhelming, but I promise it is not. It is the same tracker I used to find the source of my migraines. All it took was a small notebook, some colored pencils, and a little time after each meal or when my symptoms flared up.

Most craft stores carry small notebooks filled with plain paper. They're usually no more than a hundred or so pages, each page about the size of a postcard. In all likelihood, this is all the paper you'll need for your tracker. If you're experiencing a wide range of symptoms, you may be facing down a couple of food sensitivities. In these cases, you might want to opt for a larger notebook. This will give you room to track whether or not certain foods trigger all your symptoms or only some of them.

Once you've selected your notebook size, take a moment to think about what symptoms you're having. If you're having symptoms like general headaches, upset stomach, frequent trips to the bathroom, or skin irritation, you can use checkboxes to indicate when you experience symptoms. Simply date one page for each day and write a list of possible symptoms at the top. Then, in the middle of the page, you can track what you eat at each meal. When you experience a symptom, you can put a check next to it on your list and write down which meal you ate prior to experiencing the symptom.

If you're experiencing symptoms on a gradient, however, you might want to use a color-coding system. My biggest symptom was migraines. So, to track them, I outlined a box in heavy black ink. I would color in the box, starting at the top, with a color that matched how much pain I felt. Green meant no pain. From there the colors would fade from green to yellow to orange to red depending on my pain level. Migraines that sent me to bed in a darkened room were colored in purple.

Each time I hit a new pain level, I would make a note of whether or not I ate an hour or so before the symptom set in and what time the pain began to intensify. Over the course of a few months, I realized that I always experienced pain in direct proportion to the amount of gluten I had eaten. I would never have found my sensitivity if I hadn't tracked my pain level and what was going on when it changed.

You can adapt this system to fit nearly any symptom. When you think you have a lead, you can take the tracker to a doctor. They can more easily help you track any other side effects of your sensitivity if they have your tracker to base their tests on.

This tracker is specifically for food allergies. But you can personalize your tracker until it covers all the bases you need it to. The next section in this chapter will cover general trackers, their benefits, and how to avoid the trap of over-tracking or burning out.

Food Trackers: The Why and How

You probably know someone who uses a food tracker. And this person probably falls into one of two categories. They either rave about their food tracker and all the good it has done them. Or they complain about it and grimace every time they have to record their newest meal.

The difference in these people is not based on what they're tracking or why they're using a food tracker. More likely than not, one person is using a tracker suited to their needs while the other is not. I think we can all agree that we'd rather be the first person than the second person (even if the first person can be a bit frustrating at dinner parties). But before you can find a tracker that works for you, you will need to make sure you need a food tracker at all.

While most people would probably learn something interesting by tracking their eating habits, a detailed food tracker is going to be overkill. For the most part, you won't need to know the exact weight or quantity of your food so that you can record the calories and nutrients you take in with each meal. At most, you probably just need to write down what you eat and note serving sizes like "two spoons of mixed vegetables with butter and salt" or "half a chicken breast with barbecue sauce".

There are a few exceptions to this rule, of course. People trying to lose weight or adjust the ratios of what they eat will want to invest in a food scale and track their portions a little more closely. If you're trying to reduce your carb intake, for example, tracking your specific serving sizes will help you make sure you're making the progress you want to make.

It's important to note that, whichever group you fall into, there's no need to go out and buy an expensive planner or a gadget that comes with a meal tracking app. You can create a fully customized food tracker using a notebook or free printables found online.

The size of your tracker will depend on the amount of information you need to track. If you're just keeping a general eye on what you're eating, you can use a notebook small enough to fit in your pocket or a note-taking app on your phone. If you want to keep a more detailed log, however, you'll want something closer to a full-size notebook or printouts on full sheets of paper and kept in a special binder.

Each person's situation will be different. And this means that everyone's tracker will be different. But there are a few key features that every tracker should have. Every planner should have a separate page for each day so that you have all the room you need to track your meals with space left over to add any notes you come up with.

Your planner should also have outlined sections for each meal or snack you eat. This will keep you from getting information crossed over when you read back over your records. When you're first starting out, keep these boxes as simple as possible. Once you've gotten into the habit, however, you might want to color-code the meals or the type of food consumed in each meal.

If you're trying to make a specific change to your diet, you might also want to write the details of that change at the top of each page.

This will help you keep your goals in mind whenever you go to write down what you've eaten. Even if you slip up with one meal, reading your goals when you write down the meal should help you stay on track the next time you eat.

You might also want to include a page at the beginning of every week where you write a meal plan. Planning your meals ahead of time will help keep you on track, even if you're only pre-planning one meal each day. You can use these meal plans to write out grocery lists and make sure you leave enough time in your day to get the nutrition you need.

Food trackers can help you make amazing changes in your life. The key is to make sure that they remain a help, not a hinderance. If you find that tracking your food becomes so stressful it's affecting your relationship with food, change how you're tracking your information. You can reduce the amount of information you're writing into your log or you can skip a few days altogether. Your tracker should always, first and foremost, be a tool that helps you achieve your goals.

Diving into New Foods

As you make changes to your diet, you might find that you have to cut out foods you once relied on. My family, for example, *loved* meals based on bread and pasta. But when we discovered I couldn't eat gluten anymore, we had to drop most of our standby meals and come up with new ones.

Trying new foods can be a little daunting. And this is even more true when the new goods are intended to replace foods, you're comfortable with but can no longer eat. Thankfully, there are a few ways to take some of the sting out of the experience. There are also a few ways you can bring new foods into your life without spending a ton of money on ingredients you don't normally use.

If you have to replace an old favorite food, you can choose one of two approaches. Some people find it helpful to replace foods with alternatives that are as similar as possible. In the case of semolina pasta, which has gluten, a lot of people prefer chickpea pasta. Alternatives allow you to sub out ingredients almost one for one so your recipes don't have to change that much.

The downside of finding similar alternatives is that they might not come close enough. Pasta made from corn, for example, has a different texture and flavor than semolina pasta. It also cooks up differently so you might not be able to use the alternative in all of your recipes. Direct substitutions can also cost more, since they're sold to a niche market. If you're on a tight grocery budget, you might find your money better spent on ingredients for entirely different recipes.

This brings us to the second option. If you have recipes you can no longer make, don't look for direct substitutions. Instead, look at *why* you like that particular recipe. Is it the combination of meat and cheese? Do you like how salty the meal is? Or maybe it balances spicy and sweet at just the right level.

Once you find what specifically you like about a recipe, you can find new ones that fill the same niche but don't use the ingredients you're trying to avoid. You might even find a new favorite! This approach is especially helpful if you're trying to avoid an entire category of food.

If, for example, you've been advised to try the ketogenic diet, you have to avoid carbs. For most people, this means cutting out breads and pastas entirely. Substitutions won't reduce your carb count, but cutting out the foods entirely can leave you with some very unsatisfactory meals. Bunless burger anyone?

But if you approach these recipes by looking for things that taste the same without involving the ingredients you need to avoid, you can come up with some great alternatives. Cheeseburger casserole can be just as good as a cheeseburger. Or if you have to avoid pizza so you can cut gluten, a pizza casserole can deliver all the saucy, cheesy goodness you need with the toppings you love.

Of course, food allergies and sensitivities aren't the only reason to try new foods. Trying new things stimulates our minds. And, as discussed in chapter two, we live longer, fuller lives when our minds are active. The best part is that it is very easy to work new foods into your diet. Even if you're on a budget, there are a few ways you can explore utterly novel flavors without completely restocking your pantry with ingredients you're not familiar with.

If you want to try new foods as a way to expand your horizons, your best bet is to try the food at a restaurant before you try making it at home. This will let you try it when it's been made by people with a lot of experience. When you choose the restaurant, make sure to look at online user reviews so you find one of your best local offerings.

Trying new food is always more fun when you bring a friend. You can each get a new dish and share a little bit with each other so you get to try even more new food. If your goal is to try several new foods, you can make a special event out of it by trying one new food each month. This will let you budget for the outing as well as plan ahead so you can make the most of your evening.

When you're ready to bring a new recipe home, start with one that resembled something you know. If you know how to cook chicken, try a recipe that uses a new combination of spices. That leaves you with a minimal investment in new ingredients and a whole new world of flavor to explore.

You can also start small by trying a dessert or appetizer. There are complex options in both categories, to be sure. But most appetizers are easy when compared to entrees. Salads and soups are, generally speaking, easier as well. Desserts can be complex, but every cuisine has a few options that are simple, delicious, and – more often than not – a form of comfort food. These recipes are excellent options for people just starting out in a particular cuisine.

Trying new recipes at home is also a great reason to invite friends over. You can prepare your new dish and make an evening out of having everyone taste it. This is an excellent opportunity to share your new interests with friends. And, when you're trying to make a change in your life, combining goals like this is a great way to reduce your energy output and keep yourself motivated.

A Final Note

Food nourishes our bodies but it can do so much more than that. It can motivate you when you're learning something new. When shared with friends, it can mend relationships and strengthen those that are already in a good place. Food has long been a touchstone in every culture and it will be no different for you.

In order to get the most from your food – and the time you spend with it – you need to try and have as healthy a relationship with it as possible. Yes, comfort food is essential for most people. But it should not be your only comfort. On the flip side of that, food should not be a source of anxiety. There is no reason to feel shame or discomfort because of the food you eat. It's there to nourish your body and help you achieve your goals.

When you change the way you interact with food, you will change the way you interact with yourself and the world around you. Food is everywhere. It is in the advertising we see and it is a key motif in just about all the media we watch. There is a reason that fan-made cookbooks are so common when a franchise becomes popular.

Food connects us to other people. It lets us reach out when we don't have words and it gives people a common ground on which to meet. There is always some way to tie food into your interests, no matter what they are. Humans being the social creatures we are, crave these chances to interconnect.

And that is why the lessons you learn in this chapter – the lessons on trying new things and sharing your newfound tastes with friends – can so easily carry into the next chapter. Food is nourishment and food is one of the main foundations of society. So, let your interest in food feed the social connections in your life.

CHAPTER 5
SOCIAL CONNECTIONS

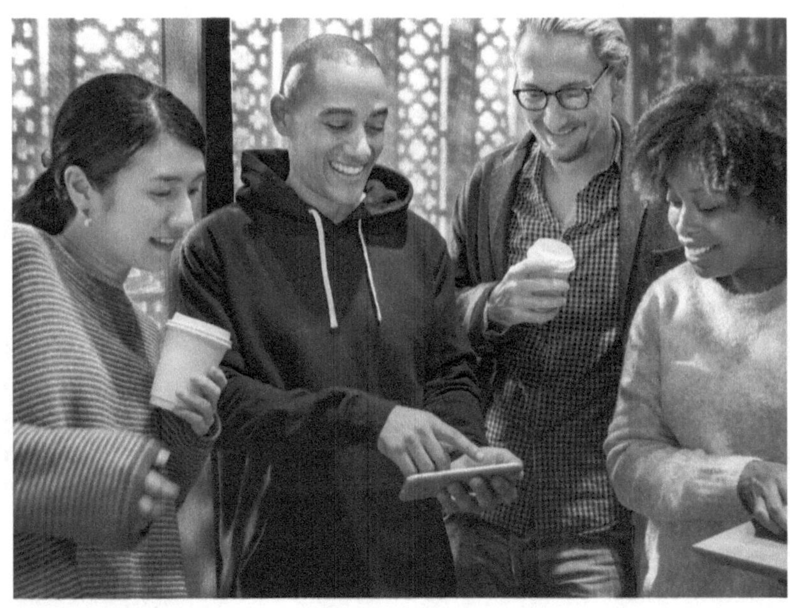

You are human. That means that you are a social creature. Some people are extremely social. Others can only handle socializing in small doses. Yet others can only comfortably socialize with people they already know or who they meet through someone they trust. Your level of social comfort doesn't change that humans are social creatures.

So, when we talk about making your life better or about prolonging your life, we have to talk about social connections. You might still be in the prime of your youth or you might have decades under your belt. But no matter your age, you need to work at building and maintaining social connections.

The "how" of socializing changes as we age. But the risks of loneliness and the importance of community never changes. This chapter will cover both the problem with loneliness as well as suggestions on countering the issue through new social connections. There is an entire section dedicated to build up those social connections, with tips to cover most phases of our lives.

If you're not the type who makes friends easily, don't flip to another chapter. This information is for you too. There are sections on using what you know to build up connections with people you're already in contact with, as well as a whole section on techniques you can use to find new social connections.

And as social as humans are, there are those among us that feel drained by intense or frequent social interactions. For those people, there is a section on how to balance the importance of being social with the necessity of caring for your own mental health and well-being.

Our lives are busy. But that is no reason not to get out and make a few friends. They can help you make the most of your life, encourage you to follow your dreams, and – according to some studies – they may even help prolong your life. Making friends might be hard. But it is a challenge that is well worth taking on.

Loneliness is All Too Common

Loneliness has been a part of human culture for as long as humans have been humans. Not all that long ago, every society on the planet consisted of small groups that were relatively close-knit. But even among these groups, there were those who feel they did not quite belong. Sometimes these people struck out to find another group they might fit better with. At other times, they stayed with the group they knew and made the best of it. But, in both cases, they still reached out to other humans.

Unfortunately, loneliness is even more rampant today. And it doesn't seem to be getting any better with the advent of social media and extreme connectivity. To be clear, I'm not about to go on an anti-technology rant. These innovations are here to stay, in some form or another. And that means we need to find ways to work them into our culture.

But there is something amiss when literally millions of people – if not billions – are at our fingertips and we still feel lonely. And I'm no sociologist, but in my experience, it has something to do with the lack of a common thread. Yes, you can reach out and comment on a music video online and get four hundred comments back within a few days. But the only thing you have in common with all those people is that you all watched the same music video.

Loneliness is best combatted when we feel a genuine connection with other people. Although you watched the same music video as all of those people, you don't know their opinions on the band. It's hard to hold a sprawling conversation over comment threads where responses can get muddled and linked to the wrong original post. It's not impossible to make friends over this medium. For some, it might even be easier than face to face interaction. But that doesn't mean it's easy.

You're not alone if you spend a lot of time online and still feel lonely. It's a common occurrence that social scientists have been studying for years. There's no clear solution in sight yet. But, for a lot of people, it helps to know that they're not the only ones experiencing this situation. They're not. You're not.

It's also important to note that feeling lonely, even when you're in a room full of people, is also possible. This usually happens when we're hiding a part of ourselves from the people around us.

It might be as silly as a guilty pleasure movie or band. Or it might be something as profoundly personal as our orientation. No matter what we're keeping to ourselves, this creates a feeling like the people around us can't really see us. Like we – our real selves – aren't even in the room with all those people.

Everyone feels lonely from time to time. Despite this, there is still some kind of cultural shame that surrounds admitting you're lonely.

So many people – men especially – are told that if they're lonely they should just keep it to themselves. They should be tough. Or, possibly worse, they're told that they're only lonely because they don't appreciate the people they already have. Neither of these statements is true.

You are not selfish because you're lonely. And you don't have to be tough. You, as a human, are wired to crave the company of others with whom you can just relax and be yourself around. People you can let down your guard for. Everyone deserves that.

As a final note on loneliness, there are times when loneliness is more than a need for companionship. If you find that you are *always* lonely or that you will feel content with a person one moment and lonely the next without anyone leaving the area, you might want to speak with someone. These are both signs of depression, among other issues.

Mental illness is not a personal failing any more than loneliness is. But it is a serious issue that you should talk to a professional about. Just as you deserve community and companionship, you deserve help when you need it.

Socializing Throughout Life

The way we make friends changes as we grow older. When we're children, it's as easy as making friends with the person whose desk is next to yours or who has the same shoes. That's a bit of an oversimplification, of course. But it's not far from the truth. Children make and break friendships very quickly.

But as we grow, both making and losing friends becomes harder. You can make friends with people in your classes when you're in high school and college. Coworkers can become friends as well. And, of course, there are parties and mixers where you can mingle with people your own age who are about to share the same classes, teachers, and school-guided events as you.

Making friends after college is a little bit harder. And that's not to say that making true friends in the midst of all these events is easy either. To help resolve some of the frustration that can come with making friends, I've gathered a few tips that have worked well for me over different periods of my life.

High School and College

It is arguably easier to make friends when you're in high school and college. Your classes force you to see the same people at set times every week. Sometimes you see them every day. These shared connections and repeated exposure are part of what social scientists now tell us to form the basis for friendships. Our minds know these people will be in a certain place at a certain time and we come to enjoy that reliability.

But not all of our classmates will mesh with our personalities. Others might take offense to part our views or interests. In both situations, no amount of repeated exposure is going to smooth out all the rough edges. Making friends in these situations requires more than being in the same place at the same time for a few months at a time.

When you're in your school days and making friends, try to find some common ground. Look for band stickers or pop culture merchandise. If you already share that interest, make a casual comment about it. Should they be interested in something you're unfamiliar with, you can ask them questions. When it comes to making friends, asking other people about themselves is a much faster route than just sharing your own views.

You can also connect with people based on the views they share in class. If someone shares an opinion that you resonate with, take a moment after class and let them know. It's a good way to let them know you're listening to them and that your opinions line up with theirs.

Extracurricular groups are also a great place to meet friends. Your options might be a little limited in high school, depending on where you live. But many colleges have student-organized groups for every interest from cultural to athletic to mythological to gaming groups. Joining these groups might seem daunting at first. But everyone in the group was the new person at some point. They know how you feel and, in many cases, will make you feel welcome.

If your school doesn't have a group that strikes your interest, you can probably start your own. Each school and university has its own unique requirements for people who want to host a group. But a quick trip to the main office or student administration building should get you a copy of the requirements. Then all you have to do is fill out the paperwork, meet the requirements, and set a date!

Starting your own group presents its own unique kind of challenge. But it also presents an amazing opportunity. When the group is smaller, you can get to know your members on a very personal level. You know that you all have a shared interest and you can build from there.

As the group grows, you'll find that you end up in more of an administrative position, but that can also have its benefits when it comes to making friends! People will come forward who want to help you run the group, which is a good indication that you have the same goals. That is an excellent basis on which to form a friendship.

When School is Done

Most of us graduate college a little bit before we turn thirty. Not all, but most. I make this distinction because the way you socialize doesn't so much change with age as it does with the places you meet people. And, because most people get out of school sometime in their mid to late twenties, this section is geared for that age range and a little bit beyond.

If you're in this age range, you probably don't have access to student groups anymore. But that doesn't mean you are out of options when it comes to finding interest-focused groups. And interest-focused groups are effective as effective after your school years as they are when you're befriending your classmates. These groups still give you a guaranteed shared interest on which you can build a solid friendship.

Finding an interest-based group near you is a little trickier when you're not in school. There are several websites that allow people to create groups based on their interests and location, which you can find by searching for your interest and the words "group near me". Any site that hosts these kinds of events will pop up as a possible search solution.

You might also have some luck with social media. Many groups create pages on the major social media websites so potential members can find them. If you're not one for generalized social media and prefer sites specifically catering to your interest, you can look there for local groups as well. These groups will sometimes have threads on message boards and so on. These allow members to post meeting times and announce whether or not they can attend specific events.

Of course, there are other ways to meet friends when you leave school. Many graduates are quick to say that making friends is harder, and that is true. But it is far from impossible. In addition to special interest groups, you might look for community events in areas near you. These can range from art walks – where you can talk to other people enjoying the fruits of local artists – to trivia and karaoke nights at your local pub, tavern, or bar. It goes without saying that you have to be at least twenty-one before you can attend the latter events.

One of the biggest obstacles you're going to come up against is your own fear. You might fear rejection or failure. You might even fear looking ridiculous when you sing karaoke or if you try talking to someone and they aren't interested. But a long time ago I learned a secret that helped with my own fear of looking ridiculous: everyone worries that they're going to look like a fool. Literally everyone. Movie stars, celebrities, politicians, people on the street.

Every single one of us feels like there is a spotlight on us all the time. In our minds, we are the center of the story because we can only really perceive things from our own point of view. But the truth of the matter is that most people aren't paying attention to you or to me. They're paying attention to themselves, the people they know, and the people who seem larger than life.

Sure, if you sing off-key into a microphone at a bar full of people, folks are going to notice. But that doesn't mean they're going to be talking about it tomorrow. They probably won't even be talking about it five minutes after your song wraps up. You're just a blip in their story, just like they're a blip in yours.

When I realized this – and learned to repeat the lesson whenever my fear got too strong – I found the courage to really put myself out there. And it can help you too. Yes, you're a footnote in their story. And that might be a hard pill to swallow because we all want to feel important. But it also means that you're free to live your story free of their judgment. They won't remember what you do unless you become one of those larger-than-life people (and even then, they'll forget the details in a few months). So, do what makes you happy.

This attitude can go a long way when you're trying to make new friends. You don't have to make a fool of yourself for people to like you. But if you're willing to try new things without looking ashamed of yourself when you make a mistake, people will see you as someone that won't judge them when *they* make a mistake. Friendships based on a shared sense of trust are the kind that last. And that's the foundation you're laying when you show you are willing to take chances and just learn from any missteps that happen along the way.

The Golden Years

However, you feel about the term "The Golden Years", you have to admit they do a good job of telling you which phase of your life this section touches on. Now, admittedly, I am not yet myself in my golden years. But I have spent quite a bit of time talking with family and friends that *have* entered this particular stage of their life. And their tips are, well, golden.

Many people in this age bracket are either retired or, largely, working with people in different stages of their lives. And while it is completely possible – and even encouraged – for people to make friends whose life experience is wildly different, there is something to be said for meeting people who have lived just as long as you have. People who, more or less, remember the same things you do and lived through the same cultural events.

To this end, there are a few things you can do that increase your odds of meeting more people you can relate to on this level. Before we move to the tips, however, it is important to touch on loneliness one more time. Not just because you might be dealing with it but because the people around you are likely dealing with it as well.

Extended periods of loneliness can cause depression, anxiety, and a whole host of other problems. And when people are suffering under the symptoms of these issues, motivation is a struggle. If you know this first-hand, I encourage you to look up the number for a hotline that you can call. There are several designed specifically for people in your age group to call so that you can talk with people who relate to what you're going through.

If you're fortunate enough not to experience these issues first-hand, you might still run into them as you try to make friends. Someone you talk to at an event might not show up again for a few weeks. You might exchange contact information with someone and not hear from them as they promised you would. When this happens, try reaching out to the other person. Even just one attempt lets the other person know you're interested in pursuing a friendship. It might be the motivation they need to connect with you and other people, bringing them out of their loneliness.

This is a bit of a low note to start our tips on, I admit. But it's an important and often overlooked fact that should be acknowledged when talking about making friends in this stage of your life. Of course, you need to get out there and meet people before you have to concern yourself with this possibility.

As with other times in your life, interest-based groups are a great way to go. You can attend a general one and meet people of all ages. Or, using the same methods that I outlined in the last section, you can find a group designed specifically for people in your age group.

These age-specific groups most often take the form of singles mixers, which can be a great way to meet prospective romantic partners as well as potential friends. If you aren't looking for romance, however, you can always limit your search to groups that focus on socializing rather than fraternizing.

One of the best things about these groups is that, in many cases, you will meet a person and the friendship will dovetail into other relationships. Someone you meet in a special interest group might invite you to their place of worship, a family dinner, or to go along with them to another group.

Many people have lost the shyness of their youth by this point in their lives and are more willing to be open with the people around them. This can lead to fast friendships forming in the space of only a few weeks. And though this might seem fast, it's actually a good thing. It leads to more open communication that, to be frank, should be common between many more people than it is.

Building Up Connections

So far, we have spent a lot of time talking about how to meet new people. But there comes a time when you have plenty of casual friends and what you really need is some idea on how to deepen your connection with some of them. This sounds daunting. And, when you make the active choice to do this, it can seem a little less than genuine. But if you honestly want to be closer with someone, making a deliberate attempt at it is the most genuine thing you can do.

And, thankfully, it's not as hard as it seems. There are several time-honored methods for turning acquaintances into fast friends. You will have to tailor the approaches to your specific friends, of course. And I give a few suggestions throughout this section on how to tailor each approach, using a few examples. But, in the end, these are people you know and want to know better. Go with what your gut tells you.

The first method is one I touched on in the last chapter. People used to say that the fastest way to a man's heart was through his stomach but, honestly, that holds true for everyone. Food has been a community-building tool for as long as people have cooked. We need food to survive and, on some level, sharing your food still seems to register as helping other people survive. Even if it's just a few cookies from your lunch at work every few days.

You don't have to cook your friends a gourmet meal, of course. And you don't have to treat them to an expensive dinner every time you hang out. In fact, if you aren't in the habit of cooking for other people, it's best to start small.

You can bake cookies or brownies and bring them to the next group meeting. If your friend has an allergy or sensitivity, this is an excellent chance to show them that you care about them. You can bake cookies for the group and then make a batch for your friend that uses alternatives for the foods they can't have. Not only will you cheer everyone up with some cookies but your friend will absolutely love that you made sure they could feel included.

If you're not part of a group, you can make some cookies and invite your friend over to hang out. Again, if they have a food sensitivity, this will be especially touching. Most people loved baked goods and enjoy hanging out with people who have treats on hand. And if your treats are tailored to your friend's needs, they will know that you thought of them when you baked the goodies.

Once you get the hang of small things like cookies, you can invite people over for dinner. Slow cookers are a great way to work on the skills you need to feed a group. The slow cooker will take care of the meat – or stew – and you can put your immediate focus on making a salad or cutting up cheese, fruit, and vegetables for a snack platter.

Most slow cooker meals are easy and, thanks to the size of most slow cookers, easily feed a whole group. You can also easily make your own slow cooker recipes by putting your favorite meat and condiment into the slow cooker with a little bit of liquid. Some things, like ranch, are definitely not suited for this cooking style. But barbecue sauce, soy sauce, and hot sauce will all simmer into the meat and give it a wonderfully deep flavor. Just be sure to stand back when you open the lid if you're using hot sauce. That steam *will* carry a serious sting and can hurt your eyes.

As easy as they are to make, slow cooker meals are usually huge crowd-pleasers. Cheesy Chicken, barbecue pulled pork, and beef stew are all slow cooker staples and there are rarely leftovers. If your slow cooker has a latched lid you can even take it with you for a group potluck, should that be where you're making your friends.

But what do you do if food isn't your strong suit? Or if it just doesn't fit the type of group, you're in, or the friends you're trying to make. In these cases, there are a few other things you can do. These tips are a little harder to implement than bringing food for the simple fact that they are not as ingrained in human culture. They are effective, nonetheless. You might just have to give them a little extra time before you try a new tactic or start seeing results.

The first way you can build up your connection with someone is asking them to do something else with you. If you typically meet in a group setting, you could ask them to check out a local shop or grab coffee sometime. You can also ask if they have an online place you can link up with them. A lot of people have blogs or video game profiles that they're happy to share with people they want to get to know better.

My next tip might sound a little counterintuitive but hear me out: ask people to help you with something. Social scientists have found that asking people for small favors – keeping an eye out for a new game expansion or going with you to an event you're too nervous to go to on your own – is even more effective in increasing friendship levels than offering to do someone a favor.

This is because asking someone to help you with something shows that you trust them. Offering to do them a favor is all well and good. But trusting them to come through for you makes them feel special. You don't want to overdo it, of course. Don't ask someone to help you move, then to wash your car, then to pet-sit your cat all in short order.

But if you ask someone to check on your cat when you're out of town overnight and then make them cookies as a thank you, it's a great way to increase your connection with them. It shows that you trust them with both your house key and your pet. Then, on top of that, you show them that you appreciate their time by making them a small gift.

There are other ways you can increase your connection with someone that relies wholly on how you met them. If you met someone at your place of worship, you can ask them to do a reading of your religious text with you. Friends you met through a book club might enjoy hearing a playlist you made based on the most recent book the group covered. And a friend from a crafting group would probably love to do a craft-along with you, where you all do the same pattern and see how your projects differ at the end.

One thing you need to remember, no matter how you choose to reach out to people, is that these people are already your friends. They already like you and enjoy spending time with you. If you're nervous about becoming closer to them, just repeat that statement to yourself: They are already my friends. At worst, they won't have much time to spend hanging out with you. At best, they have wanted to get closer to you as well and just didn't know how to go about it.

Earlier I said that everyone thinks they are at the center of the story because we can only see things from our point of view. And that is certainly true. But there is another side to it as well. When you look at other people, you are seeing the polished exterior. You can't see their inner turmoil or their self-doubt. And that means that they can't see yours. So, when you're nervous and you think your friend isn't, remember that you can't see in their mind. There's every chance they have the same thoughts you do.

Balancing Socializing and Self-Care

Humans are social animals. We crave contact with other humans. But, for some of us, there are limits. The limit might be on how often we can socialize, or for how long. For some people, the limit is on the type of interactions they're comfortable with. And as important as socializing is, it is just as important that you honor your boundaries.

There is a fine line between pushing yourself to try new things and pushing yourself so far out of your comfort zone that you experience negative reactions. If you're not used to socializing you will probably find it tiring to be out with people for hours at a time. But as long as an evening of self-care recharged your batteries, that's a boundary you should push.

If, on the other hand, you end up shaking or experiencing panic attacks because you can't handle being in a large crowd, steer clear of that boundary. When – or if – you choose to address that issue, you should do it with the help of a professional. Certain issues are best handled by someone with extensive training. And anything that induces panic attacks certainly belongs on that list.

When you're pushing your boundaries – and especially if panic attacks are a risk for you – you need to learn your cues before you dive into trying new things. Some people find that their breathing becomes shallow when they're nearing the edge of their tolerance level. Other people experience clammy skin. And, for many people, talking becomes much less appealing. Learn your body's specific cues and have an exit strategy. Even something as simple as "I have to call my grandmother for her birthday" is a good way to dart out and get some air or leave the event entirely.

If you already have a close friend and are looking to make more, you can ask your friend to attend events with you. Depending on how well you know your friend, they might know your cues already. They can let you know when you're starting to shut down and help you get out of there without anyone knowing why you're leaving.

Some people feel bad when they leave an event early. But, if it's between leaving early and maintaining a comfortable mental health balance, you should always leave early. You can always come back to the next event when you're feeling better. Taking care of yourself and your mental health is absolutely vital to making friends. And meeting new people should never come at the expense of your own well-being.

A Final Note

When you're reading through all of these tips, it can be easy to lose sight of what they are all for. You are reading this book because you want to live a longer, healthier life. Making friends is part of that. As we age, loneliness finds it easier to slip into our lives. And it seems like every year, more social scientists tell us that feeling lonely or cut off can shorten our life spans.

If you want to live a longer life, you improve your odds by making friends. It can be messy and uncomfortable. But it is well worth the time you invest. Even casual friends get you out of the house, stimulate your mind, and give you someone to connect with. Close friends offer a sense of security and comfort. And intimate friends allow you to completely be yourself without fear of isolation.

But as important as friends are for prolonging our lives, the quality of our friends determines if they improve the health of our lives. Go out and make friends, of course. But be sure that they share your values. Do not settle for people who encourage unhealthy behaviors just because they will be your friends. This might seem silly to say, but loneliness can make people do silly things.

Throughout this book, I have encouraged you to develop compassion toward yourself. When you are out there making friends, make sure you keep your self-talk compassionate and kind. Getting to know new people can be tough. It's even tougher if you're coming from a place of loneliness. Just remember that the effort you put in now will help improve the quality and length of your life.

CHAPTER 6

SELF-CARE

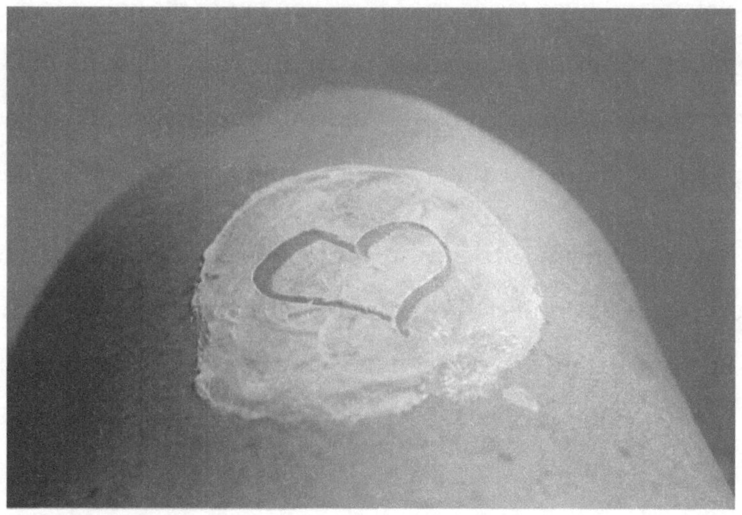

Self-care, as a term, became popular as the Millennial generation aged into full adulthood. But that does not mean that the concept is new. People have been carrying out acts of self-care throughout history. And despite appearances on social media, self-care does not have to include a spa day or expensive chocolates.

When you're trying to live a longer, healthier life, you have to make some changes. And so far, we have stayed together through a whole litany of changes from diet and exercise to making friends to changing the way you talk to yourself. But, at the root of it all, this is about you. Not the changes you're making or the place you want to go. All of this is about your wellbeing and your happiness.

So, with this in mind, it seems fitting that the last chapter of this book will cover self-care. We will cover what self-care is (and what it isn't). From there we will move into several kinds of self-care from the mental to the physical and then to the spiritual. While both physical and mental self-care are very specific categories, I want to take a moment to touch on spiritual self-care. Because this book is written for people of many faiths, I will use general suggestions and terms so that you can choose the type of self-care the works for you and your faith.

Finally, the last section of this chapter will offer daily self-care ideas that you can piece together to form your perfect daily self-care ritual. As with all things, remember to talk to yourself with compassion as you're working through this chapter. There is no shame in spending some time on yourself, just as there is no shame in having been unable to do so before now.

Self-care is about compassion. It is about loving yourself inside and out. And, because you care for yourself, you will have a better chance of reaching the goals you have set for yourself. I ask that you take your time on this chapter, even more so than the others. If something in these pages sparks a new idea that suits you better, by all means, write it down and use it. Follow your instincts and do what works best for your life and your needs. In this way, you can live your fullest life.

Self-Care: Fact and Fiction

Before we get into self-care suggestions, I want to spend some time talking about what self-care is. And, just as importantly, I want to cover the things that self-care is not. For some readers, this section might seem obvious. But, for some people, self-care has come to mean utter self-indulgence. And, because of this, they do not see how vital real self-care is. For them and for other people.

Self-care, at its most simple, is doing things that make you feel refreshed. It is also doing things that you do not usually have the motivation for, but impact your quality of life. The term became popular when Millennials – one of the first generations to speak openly and frankly about mental health issues and their symptoms – aged into adulthood. When this happened, people began to admit that certain daily tasks were difficult to carry out when they struggled with anxiety or depression.

This led to other people admitting that increased workloads, advancing age, and other social pressures also made it hard for them to match the ideal that they aimed for. As these admissions became more popular, so did the idea that we as a society should have more compassion for ourselves and for people who might struggle to hit all the marks, we think we're supposed to.

What this really amounted to was putting a new name on an old concept. This concept has been called many things over the years.

Terming is "self-care" is just putting a finer point on an idea that was otherwise talked about in broad terms. It's been called a "spa day", a "girls' weekend", or a "boys' night". It's a time when it is socially acceptable to focus on yourself and your friends. Doing only what you like to do and not worrying about everything else.

Unfortunately, the term has been tapped into by people with an eye toward marketing. Cosmetic companies, shaving companies, and even car companies have used the idea of self-care to promote the idea that people have to spend money to take care of themselves. On the one hand, this makes sense. The job of marketing people is to sell us things. But it also gives the wrong impression about what self-care is.

Yes, self-care can be getting yourself a new car. But only if it reduces your overall stress level. If your current car barely runs and you're never sure if you can get to work because of it, then invest in a new car. But that isn't a free pass to buy the newest sports car or go wild with the amenities. Do whatever reduces your stress level and helps you breathe easier. *That* is self-care.

Self-care can also be turning your phone off for an hour when you're feeling overwhelmed or make yourself turn off the TV and write out a meal plan for the next week so you know what you're making for dinner and the groceries in your fridge won't go bad. Both of these things can help you live a longer, healthier life by bringing down your stress level and making sure you support yourself.

If you have ever heard the term "self-care" only to groan and roll your eyes, you're not alone. A lot of people have gotten the wrong impression. The only time they see someone talk about self-care are celebrities who buy expensive clothes or marketing campaigns promoting the newest luxury item. But I promise you, it is so much more than that.

Self-care is compassion. It is compassion for yourself. And, in more distant fashion, it is compassion for the people around you. When you support yourself – when you take the time to check in with your own well-being – you are a better friend. You're a better partner, parent, coworker, and lover. Your compassion spills over from yourself to other people. When more people do this, it can create a ripple effect that changes so much more than indulging in a box of chocolates can.

Even if you're still not entirely sure about the idea of self-care, I ask that you take some time and try it for yourself. Look through the suggestions in this chapter and try a few out for yourself. Even small changes that focus on your well-being can have a huge impact on the quality and duration of your life.

Mental Self-Care

Since self-care started with the mental health awareness movement, it seems fitting that the first tips in this chapter focus on your mental well-being. Many of these tips are for general use but may be particularly useful if you have a history of depression or anxiety. You may also find these tips useful if, even without mental health issues, you have an extremely stressful schedule.

Many of these tips, in this section and in others, are focused on making your life easier. I have included one or two tips for treating yourself. But, for the most part, self-care should be about reducing your stress level and making your life easier. To that end, these tips are meant to help you organize your life and arrange things so that, when you're not actively engaged in self-care, you can still reap its benefits.

Set a Schedule

This might not seem like much of a tip. But humans crave routine more often than they crave novelty. Yes, we like new things. But our brains also like it when they know what to expect. And that is why a schedule is so important.

Self-help gurus and lifestyle speakers like to talk about making a hard and fast schedule that accounts for every minute of your day. Even if it's a block schedule that breaks your day into chunks, there are still hard and fast times when you do certain things. This works for some people. But for a lot of people – those with mental health issues, those with kids, and those with a variable work schedule for example – this simply doesn't work. So, to counter this, I propose only scheduling one or two hard and fast times every day.

Having only one or two hard schedule points that you must abide by creates a framework that you can build the rest of your day around. The two easiest to set, for the vast majority of people, are the time you wake up and the time you go to sleep.

Setting these two points as hard and fast times has a two-fold benefit. Your brain knows what to expect every single day and your body can get into a solid sleep rhythm. It knows exactly how much rest it is going to get so it sends its energy cues accordingly. As I mentioned in the chapter on diet and nutrition, hunger is usually our body's way of saying when it needs energy. You can learn to predict those cues with a little more accuracy when you get the same amount of sleep every night.

Now, you might toss and turn when you first lay down. Or you might hit the snooze button a few times when you wake up. And when you first try to implement this change, that will be an extremely tempting option. But over time you'll set a really solid sleep rhythm that your body signals you to follow, even when you're not paying attention.

You can also try setting a specific dinner time. Not a time for every meal, just a time for dinner. This is especially helpful if you struggle with eating too late in the day. By setting a hard and fast dinner time, you can plan your bedtime accordingly.

Even with just this one tip, you can see the way self-care takes one action and creates a web of reactions. If you go to bed at the same time every night, you don't have to pay so much attention to other things going on at that time. You know you're going to be in bed and you know you don't want to be disturbed. All you have to focus on is laying down and pacing yourself through deep breathing until you fall asleep. Incidentally, this is also a great time to practice the deep breathing exercises from chapter one.

If setting a hard point in your schedule appeals to you, there are ways you can make a treat out of it. You can download a pretty alarm app to your device. There are many on the market that use music, pictures, and even animations to bring a certain aesthetic to bear each time you turn an alarm on or off.

You can also create a small, indulgent routine around the point in your schedule. If you want to eat dinner at the same time every night, you can set a pretty place setting for yourself or light a nice-smelling candle that only burns for the duration of your meal. For those who want to try setting an alarm for bed, you can select a book of poems and read one each night before bed. Or you can use a sweet-smelling spray on your pillows that you only use at night. There are countless ways you can bring a touch of indulgence to this one simple act that can create much-needed stability in your day.

Plan Your Meals

I could write an entire book on the benefits of planning your meals. And some people have! But many of these books build meal planning up into a huge process that covers every meal, preparing meals ahead of time, and even grocery shopping with as many coupons as possible. All of this is useful! But if you're working on reducing your mental stress, it can be too much.

When you're planning your meals with self-care in mind, try focusing your plans on your biggest meal. For my family, this is dinner. I started out by planning our dinners a week in advance. From there I moved to two weeks, and then a month. When I sat down to plan, I used a whiteboard with a calendar on it. Each meal was chosen based on what my family had planned that day and who was slated to cook. It was a simple system that took a huge weight off our shoulders every day.

Try this method and see if it works for you. To make it even easier, you can write down a list of meals or recipes that you or your family thoroughly enjoy. You can then plug these into your meal plan calendar so you don't have to find new recipes each time. This isn't a new concept, of course. Taco Tuesday had to start somewhere. And though it can seem boring, knowing what you're coming home to after a long day can also be comforting.

Adding a little luxury to this task isn't hard. You can invest in a pack of whiteboard markers in every color of the rainbow. With these, it's easy to color-code your calendar to match holidays, events, or even just your mood! You can also choose a new recipe once or twice a month that might otherwise be outside of your tastes or your budget. You can even grab a frozen pizza to use if the recipe doesn't turn out to be a hit!

Physical Self-Care

Many of my suggestions for physical self-care fall into the realm of things that some people consider obvious. They are things that will help you stay in better health over time but that you may struggle within the moment. Things like hygiene care and following your food restrictions are hard to do at the moment, particularly if you have a lot on your plate. But there are ways to make them a little bit easier.

Make a Hygiene Appointment

Some people have absolutely no trouble motivating themselves to shower every day, brush and floss their teeth between meals, and do whatever steps are necessary to keep their hair healthy. This suggestion is not for those people, though they are welcome to use it! For a lot of people, hitting all these marks in a day is a struggle. They get caught up with work or errands or they're just too exhausted to put in the effort. People with chronic health issues – both mental and physical –

especially struggle with this because they already put so much effort into managing their health.

If you struggle with these tasks, you are far from alone. And there is no shame in admitting that taking care of yourself in this way is a struggle for you. But once you admit that it is a struggle, it is time to work on it. Luckily, working on it can take the form of self-care.

Instead of beating yourself up for not getting a shower in or for not using the proper pillowcase for your hair, use the compassionate thinking exercise from chapter one. From there, make a hard appointment to check this task off tomorrow.

Using the suggestions from the previous section in this chapter, try a few alarm apps until you find one that really motivates you. From there, find some small incentive to help motivate you. If your favorite scent is lemon, buy a bar of lemon-scented soap or get some lemon spray to treat your linens with. Finally, if you put a lot of pressure on yourself to complete this task, give yourself a little break afterward. Do not schedule anything for ten or twenty minutes after the task is supposed to be done. Instead, take this time to read or play a game. Give your mind a chance to rest while it is congratulating itself on ticking a box you struggle with.

This tip can apply to just about anything. If you struggle to remember to brush, find a toothbrush in a color you like or look online for toothpastes in different flavors. If laundry is hard for you, get an audiobook from your local library and only play it when you're working on your laundry. Both of these options will add a little bit of luxury to the task without countering the positive changes you're trying to make. And, with options like audiobooks, you can stimulate your mind while you're taking care of your body!

Make it Fun

Taking care of your body is, let's face it, kind of boring. Our bodies are commonplace, at least to us. And, for most people, tasks like working out can be absolute drudgery. But there are ways to make it fun. And tapping into these options can make it much easier for you to hit the goals you're striving toward.

If you're trying to get in more exercise, look at fitness games. There are several apps that use different storytelling motifs to encourage your physical activity level. These apps count your steps or use the camera on your phone and track exercise reps. They then use this information to reward you with in-game items and events. It might seem silly to some people. But, for others, the storytelling aspect makes exercising enjoyable enough that they are able to make a habit of it.

For those who crave a little more whimsy, you can tap into an old childhood favorite and make a sticker chart. You can either print one off the internet or create your own. Then, using stickers or stamps, you can track your progress. When you reach a certain level, you can reward yourself with something you otherwise would not indulge in.

Is this a bit juvenile? Possibly, depending on how you look at it. But is it effective and fun? Yes, absolutely! It taps into the nostalgia of childhood while blending our brain's need for both routine and novelty. And, as an added bonus, your reward doesn't have to be expensive. Yes, you can reward yourself with something a little pricey if you want to. But you can also reward yourself with video games, inviting a friend over for dinner, or checking out some sightseeing in a nearby locale you have been meaning to visit.

With this particular tip, it can be hard to find ways to incorporate a little luxury. Nobody looks good in the middle of a workout, no matter what the magazines say. We all make funny faces, turn funny colors, and sweat. It's not a good look, but it is a necessary one. The luxury, however, can come afterward. Invest in a nice shower caddy to take to the gym. Or buy a bath sheet – a giant bath towel that is incredibly soft to the touch – to wrap up in when you've cleaned yourself off.

If you're opting for a sticker chart, you can use thick paper and beautiful stamps to track your progress. Nobody says your sticker charts have to look like they did in grade school. Find one that uses calligraphy instead of Comic Sans. Buy stickers that match your general aesthetic. Incorporate the chart into a journal or scrapbook. Make it as attractive as you want so that you're working hard to get back to it as often as possible.

Spiritual Self-Care

Spiritual self-care is, as odd as it may sound, the most personal of all self-care categories. All self-care is personal, it is the nature of the act. But our spiritual lives are all one-of-a-kind. Two people can share the same religion and have vastly different personal lives. And that makes it a little hard to give suggestions on. There are a few things you can do, however.

Set a Date

Modern life is busy. And that can mean we don't get to spend as much time on our spiritual lives as we would like. But, as with everything else that we don't have time for, there is a way to counter that. Set a date. Set a hard date written on your calendar and put it into your phone. Use the same type of apps suggested in previous sections and find an alarm that really gets you moving.

When your alarm goes off, turn off all distractions. No TV, no music, no phone if you can manage it. Just you and whatever materials are used in your spiritual practice. Even five minutes in this environment can alleviate the stress you feel when you feel that you've neglected your spiritual commitments.

If you have a fairly stable schedule, you can set this date every week. Making a habit of it will take some of the stress out of the situation because you know where you're supposed to be. You can make the process by finding a candle or type of incense that you enjoy and only burning it when you're working on your spiritual practice. You can also invest in some nice notebooks and pens to take notes if that applies to your practice.

Make it Personal

Yes, our spiritual self-care is the most personal of self-care options. But it is also one that, in many cultures, we feel pressured to share. The reality is that we don't have to. Not really. And, to that end, you should take the time to make your spiritual practice as personal as possible.

If you use a spiritual text, find a copy in a font size and layout that is pleasing for you. You can most likely find carrying cases and covers that will fit the text and give it an outward aesthetic that you find soothing or attractive. You can also use notebooks, pens, highlighters, and stickers to take notes on your text and make them as personalized as possible.

In addition to all of this, you need to set aside time when you can be alone to pursue your spiritual needs. Spending time with other people in spiritual pursuits can be enriching and uplifting. But you also need to take the time to pursue your spiritual path on your own, where

you can do what feels natural without having to explain it to anyone
but yourself.

Daily Self-Care Suggestions

Self-care is very helpful, even when done sporadically. But doing
small acts of self-care every day can help reduce your overall stress level
and make it easier to accomplish your goals. These small suggestions
can be taken all together or you can pick and choose those that most
fit your needs.

Lay It Out

This is a small tip that appears in nearly every self-help book. And
for good reason. It is a small act that can make a world of difference. If
there is something you struggle to do, layout the things you need and
then come back to it. Brushing your teeth is an excellent example for
this tip.

For people who struggle to brush your teeth before bed, layout
your toothbrush and toothpaste right after dinner. Go on about your
day. Now, when you go to bed, your toothbrush, toothpaste, and floss
will all be waiting for you. It is much harder to skip over the task when
all your tools are staring at you.

This tip also works for things that might be more of an indulgence
than something you struggle with. If, for example, you want to read

more, you can set your book on your bed, propped up on your pillow. Every time you go into your room, the book on your pillow will remind you that you need to read. And, when you go to get in bed, you have to move the book so it is already in your hands. As a bonus, this might even motivate you to head to bed a little sooner each night so you have more time to read.

Plan Ahead

Decision Fatigue is a very real issue that affects all of us every day. We're bombarded with so many choices – most of which are basically choosing between two or three things that are similar – that it saps our willpower and our energy. Planning a few things out ahead of time will cut down on the number of things you have to spend your energy on, leaving you more focus on the things that matter.

You don't have to plan every meal or plan out your days. But if you know what you're having for dinner tomorrow night, you can go about your day knowing what you're doing for the evening. Or if you set out your clothes the night before, you don't have to stare down a closet full of clothes. Some people even choose to take this a step further and limit their wardrobe to a few choices that they cycle through so it's even easier to lay out their outfits.

Keep it Tidy

You don't have to live in a barren white room to have a tidy home. But a lot of visual input can make an already stressful day even worse. This is not to say that your knick-knacks or favorite collectible are visual clutter. If they're well taken care of or arranged, they can be a form of art.

But if you have stacks of papers all over your room that you don't have any purpose for, get rid of them. Organize the apps on your phone or reduce the number of icons on your home screen. Try and make your bed in the morning so that you can look at your bed and see a tidy space where you will be able to rest.

All of these things take energy but they also give you mental space to breathe. You can come home after a busy day and know that you're going to find at least a few places of complete calm in your home. And that you won't be bombarded with a million icons, apps, colors, and designs when you use your devices.

Simplify Your Commitments

This tip might prove to be the most difficult. But it is also one that made the most difference in my life. When you're feeling overwhelmed, try to simplify the things that you're committing your energy to. I touched on this in chapter one with the centering exercise. But this specific tip goes beyond visualization. It requires concrete, real-world action.

Some commitments such as family, work, and close friendships, are not things you can cut out of your life. But there are probably a dozen or so smaller commitments that you could remove from your life, even if only temporarily, without causing any real damage.

Start with the apps on your phone. You don't need to have a profile on every social media site. And, if you have a profile, it doesn't need to be updated every day. You can assign different apps to different days and, if you choose, use scheduling features to spread out when your posts go public.

On a similar note, nobody can do everything. So, if you're trying to keep a daily journal, learn a new language, follow a cleaning schedule, change your diet, and attend classes on top of a dozen other things, you're spreading yourself too thin. Instead of keeping detailed journal entries, try doing bulleted lists of your thoughts. Or you can just free-write for twenty minutes and write down whatever comes to mind. And that is if you don't want to drop the journaling entirely.

There is a lot of social pressure to use every minute of your day doing something new or productive. But that is an unhealthy pursuit that we just can't keep up with. You need to give your time mind to rest when it isn't in a REM cycle. So, if you need to uninstall your language learning app, do it without feeling any shame. Try making one change at a time instead of implementing everything all at once. And go easy on yourself if you miss a few days in your cleaning schedule – or if you only manage to follow one day of the schedule in any given week.

Get Rid of Guilty Pleasures

Of course, this doesn't mean you should stop enjoying the things you currently call your guilty pleasures. Far from it. Instead of cutting those things from your life, cut the guilt instead. The idea of guilty pleasures hinges on the concept that we should be ashamed of things we like if they're not popular. Bands that people make fun of, franchises that are overplayed. Even cartoons that are fun and harmless get thrown into the category of "guilty pleasure" if you enjoy them and you're over the age of ten.

As long as you're not hurting anyone, why should you feel guilty for enjoying something? The answer is that you shouldn't. So, take the guilt out of your guilty pleasures and keep the pleasure. You don't have to broadcast your interests if you'd rather keep them to yourself. But you don't have to hide them away either.

You might be surprised to see who shares your interests. Friends you thought might judge you may even turn out to be fans as well! There are whole groups based on the concept of watching bad movies just for the enjoyment of it. And if a franchise is overplayed, there's likely a reason for it!

Life, even a long life, is too short to worry about what other people will think of you. Acknowledging this won't magically make your anxiety go away, of course. And even the bravest among us feels self-doubt now and then. But reminding yourself that you are fully entitled to enjoy your pleasures without "guilt" added to the front may help you remember to value your opinion of your interests more than someone else's. Better yet, you can trust your own judgment more than some hypothetical person that isn't even there to judge you. Life has enough stress. The things you enjoy shouldn't be part of that.

A Final Note

Self-care might not be widely understood. But it is wildly important. It can help you reduce the stress in your life. This, in turn, helps you redirect your energy to the places it should really be. Like helping you follow your goals and your dreams. This is particularly important when you're trying to change your life for the better.

Change is never easy. It doesn't matter if the change is one you choose or one that is foisted upon you. And the bigger the change, the harder it is to implement. That is why so many sections in this book focus on small changes that balloon into larger impacts. And it is why many of the sections in this book overlap or build on one another. So that you have as many tools as possible to help you get where you're trying to go.

Self-care is just one more tool, like all the rest. It can set an excellent foundation or shore up one you've already built. Despite what some think, it is not an excuse to give yourself whatever you want or to shirk all your responsibilities. Instead, it is a chance. It is a chance to narrow your focus until you can do one thing that's been weighing on your mind.

The one thing might be cleaning up a room of your house or making a call you've been putting off. You might choose to finish a book you have had lying around for a while or to watch a movie that you've had queued for ages. It doesn't matter if you use your self-care skills to do things you normally struggle to do or if you use them to add something new and inspiring to your life.

So long as you're using your self-care methods to improve your life, you're using them properly. Proper self-care will spill over into every area of your life. You'll see the results in your improved energy levels and your reduced sense of stress. On a chemical level, you should even see a reduction in your cortisol levels. Which, as we covered early on in the book, can cause widespread damage if left unchecked.

You picked up this book because you wanted to live a longer, healthier life. You were searching for ways to improve the way you live and how you approach the world. It is my sincere hope that you found what you're looking for. No one book is going to give you all the answers. But with the tips in these pages, I sought to give you a foundation on which you could build.

Remember to start slow, with one big change you want to implement. You can always add more later, once you have the current change well in hand. If you go too big too fast, you can always scale back. If this happens, remember to show yourself compassion. Every change is a chance to learn and a chance to grow. The only real failure is the failure to try. So, try. Try and make the changes, try to reach your dreams. You have the tools. And you're worth the effort.

CONCLUSION

Thank you for making it through to the end of *Live Longer and Healthier: Ways to Live a Good Life*. I hope it was informative and able to provide you with all of the tools you need to achieve your goals and make the changes that you want to see in your life.

The next step is to apply the suggestions in this book and go at the pace that best suits your needs. Follow the passions you discovered in the learning chapter, practice the compassionate thinking you practiced in chapter one, and implement the self-care techniques you picked out from the final chapter. You have a long, rich life ahead of you. Go out and make the most it with compassion and purpose.

Finally, if you found this book useful in any way, a review on Amazon is always appreciated!

DESCRIPTION

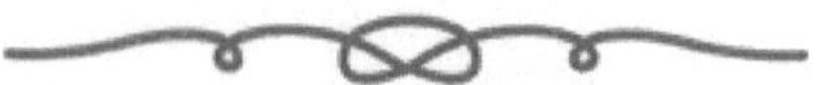

Life is short. Chances are, you want to make the most of it. This book is designed to help you do just that. Inside this book are tried and tested tips intended to help you make lasting changes in your life. Written with an emphasis on compassion and patience, this is not your typical self-help book. Each chapter is written with an eye on the specific challenges you face when you enact change in your life.

Physical fitness, nutrition, mental health and more. All of that can be found inside this book. From changing the way you think about yourself to changing the way you approach the world, *Live Longer and Healthier* has something for everyone.

Broken down into six chapters, the book covers changing your internal monologue, diving into new worlds of learning, changing the way you interact with your body, taking control of your nutrition, meeting new friends, and caring for yourself in lasting, meaningful ways. The following are just a few of the tips found in these pages

- *Talk to your with compassion* – everyone makes mistakes, especially when they are trying to change their lives. Most of us aren't taught to react to our missteps with compassion. This book will walk you through how to do just that

- *Explore your passions* – Nobody can learn everything, as much as fun as that would be. But that does not mean that we should ever stop learning. Keep your mind sharp by exploring new worlds and new ideas. And the chapter on learning offers several writing exercises to help you narrow your focus. Or, if you do not know what you want to study, there are writing exercises to help you find your passion.

- *Understand Nutrition* – Food doesn't have to be a source of anxiety. And nutrition shouldn't be a mystery. Inside this book, you will find practical tips designed to help you find out what nutrition does for your body and how to get the nutrients you need.

- *Give Self-Care a Chance* – There has been a lot of buzz about self-care. But despite that, a lot of people still don't know what it is. Check out this book chapter on self-care to demystify the concept. In addition, you'll find several suggestions for mental, physical, and even spiritual self-care.

It can be hard to change your life. But *Live Longer and Healthier: Ways to Live a Good Life* seeks to make it a little bit easier. There are suggestions in this book for everyone. From people who have yet to start the changes the way to see to people who are stuck on where to go next. Inside you will find grounding and centering techniques and guided meditations, self-care tips, and a host of other tools that you can bring to bear on your own life.

Don't wait to reach for the life you want to have. Life is short and you deserve to live the best life possible, every day. Start your journey today, with *Live Longer and Healthier: Ways to Live a Good Life.*

www.ingramcontent.com/pod-product-compliance
Lightning Source LLC
Chambersburg PA
CBHW031125250726
48655CB00002B/517